Futureproof

Futureproofing

If you can imagine it, it will happen.
If you can't – you're out of it

Roy Lilley

with a Foreword by
Professor Peter Cochrane
Head of Advanced Applications
British Telecom

THE RADCLIFFE PRESS
OXFORD AND NEW YORK

The Radcliffe Press
18 Marcham Road, Abingdon, Oxon OX14 1AA, UK

Radcliffe Medical Press, Inc.
141 Fifth Avenue, New York, NY 10010, USA

The Radcliffe Press is an imprint of Radcliffe Medical Press Ltd

British Library Cataloguing in Publication Data

A catalogue record for this book is available from the British Library.

ISBN 1 85775 136 1

Library of Congress Cataloging-in-Publication Data is available.

Typeset by Acorn Bookwork, Salisbury

... Aim: to develop a knowledge and understanding of the environment within which business activity takes place and the way in which changes in that environment influence business behaviour.

Extract from: Information Technology and Business Studies GCSE syllabus for 14 year olds

... For a system to preserve its integrity and survive, its rate of learning must at least match the rate of change in its own environment.

Ross Ashby's 'law of requisite variety', 1958

Dedication

For Linda, who has so far managed to persuade me I do have a future ...

Buy this book and what are you getting?

The ramblings of a deranged mind? Certainly! A collection of statistics, facts and figures that may come in useful one day? Yup! Some good ideas about how to run organizations? Probably! Some personal opinions on how to run the world? Definitely! A lot of stuff to make you think? Without doubt!

This book is anecdotal, provocative, rambling and a weight off my chest!

This book is a white knuckle ride. It drills down into what we are doing now, and comes up in the future to see what comes next. The book is a commentary and a clarion call and an invitation to see round corners.

There are a lot of questions on the pages and some answers. Some of the questions are not answered, because they can't be. That's the way it is. You just need to know what's lurking out there and to decide if you can beat it, take a different route, or simply roll over and play dead.

Statistics, numbers and sources

He uses statistics like a drunken man uses lamp posts – for support rather than illumination
Anon.

The statistics, numbers and ideas in this book have been culled from all kinds of sources. Academics, professionals, journalists, magazines, newspapers, books, statistical reports, saloon bars and the back of fag packets.

As I did not set out to write an academic work, I haven't let the text get bogged down in endless small print and references. The main ones, those that form the basis of the charts and diagrams, are cited. All the other facts and figures come from published government data or other official sources.

Contents

Foreword

In 1946 the author of this book and I were born within a few days of each other whilst the inventors of the transistor were still doing their seminal work. Only 14 years later silicon integrated circuits (chips) started to double their density every 12 months. This exponential growth continues today, with technology feeding technology and computers becoming 1000 times more powerful every ten years. At this rate of progress we might expect super-computers to equal the human brain by 2015. Such machines will profoundly affect our species and civilization as more compact versions will be on our desk by 2025, and may be wearing us by 2030. Moreover, these machines will be linked by optical fibre, the ultimate superhighway, to realize a world of instant gratification – information, services and experience on demand.

Making predictions is a tricky business and it is easy to be wrong, but my experience has been that the future arrives earlier than expected, and often without warning. I do not know how accurate the above picture is, but I do know the rate of progress is now such that I no longer worry about dying, but I do worry about dying before my PC is proud of me! If you are sceptical, or even totally disbelieving about such predictions, then read this book! Even if you are already convinced – you should still read this book! It will give you a new perspective; a broad framework of past, present and soon events, not through the eyes of a technologist, but through the eyes of a man who worries about the implications of change.

This book conveys the excitement and scope of change that we have already experienced and may expect in the coming decades. The technology and consequences cited are wide ranging and include the telegraph, television, atomic bomb, space race, micro-electronics, health care, shopping, intelligent houses, crime … and the way we work and live. It warns of our growing dependence on technology and need to continually adapt and change in an increasingly chaotic world.

Our technological progress is like a ratchet, it only goes in one direction! We can never go back, we can never reverse the trends unless we are prepared to pay a terrible price. To feed, clothe and look after the well-being of the near six billion population of planet earth requires high-technology and continual change. If we were to merely switch off the computers and communications network that have become the nervous system of this planet, most of us would be starving in a matter of weeks.

A modern bakery no longer has a baker, it has a computer with an artificial intelligence system that controls bread production in quantities and to a quality that we could not match. Without telecommunications there would be no way of ordering and despatching the raw materials to the bakery, or delivering the final product – bread. This is indicative of all human activity. We now have a total dependence on technology, and so we had better get it right! Should such a view engender worry and fear? I think not, for how many of us could successfully hunt down, kill and skin a rabbit? By and large, those are skills that we have long lost, along with the ability to make wagon wheels and many other artefacts on which we are very strongly dependent. Just 20 years ago many of us could lift the hood of a car and do repairs, today we just wouldn't bother, they have become far too complex with integrated engine management systems and more electronics in their control and instrumentation than used in the first Lunar Lander. Even humans are now being infiltrated by silicon technology to restore hearing through electronic links to the auditory nervous system. Early experiments bridging a severed spinal column with chips have restored momentary feeling. In one spectacular case, the movement in the hand of a paralysed victim was restored by an integrated circuit embedded under the skin. Artificial hearts are common place and soon an artificial pancreas will be with us, along with many more piece parts. This is great technology!

In contrast, some technology and change is truly unlovable! But society has the ability to steer and choose the overall direction. The real worry is not the technology, but the people who use and control it – and that has to be all of us! It is fashionable in some quarters to be openly ignorant of how things work. You often hear people emphasizing the market, regulation, competition, political considerations and decrying the existence of technology. This is dangerous, technology is tricky stuff, and we have to understand. The reality is, that long after the politicians and managers are dead and forgotten, the technology will still be there, still be remembered, still promoting change. Our job, as individual members of society, is to marshal the technology, use and steer it as if we are going to live forever.

For thousands of years mankind's journey has been like walking across the Sahara desert. The sand (a rather appropriate metaphor for technology as we use it to make optical fibre) shifted slowly so we could walk with reasonable certainty. In the past few decades these sands have started to move faster, and we have to learn to run, or we will fall over. Soon we will have to invent a hover craft (a metaphor for a new technology necessary to augment our 'wet ware' – biological brain) and learn to skim the surface instead of planting our feet on it. Reading this book will prepare you for the journey, and may even help you to run.

Professor Peter Cochrane
Martlesham Heath
Ipswich, UK
30 July 1995

Introduction

I have been speaking, gossiping and generally banging on about the subject of **Futureproofing** – what we can do to prepare ourselves for an uncertain future – all over the place, in the UK, Europe and the USA for the past four years.

My aim has been to awaken managers, entrepreneurs and anyone who will listen to the fact that the world is changing. I don't mean change in the evolutionary sense – little by little, imperceptibly, giving us a chance to adapt – but in an accelerating way. Faster and faster, spinning like a spiral. Fundamental and structural changes, leaving those who are unprepared, behind.

I don't believe it's possible for people working in modern organizations and responsible for taking major decisions, to play their part without really understanding what is going on around them.

Many members of the audiences I have spoken to have asked me for a copy of the slides I use. This book may go some way to being an apology to all those folk to whom I promised to send them, for never having got around to doing it. It also serves as a thank-you to them for their interest and support.

Roy Lilley
Surrey, UK
June 1995

CHAPTER ONE

Permanent white water

Trust no future, howe'er pleasant!
Let the Past bury its dead!
Act, – act in the living Present!
Heart within, and God o'erhead!
Longfellow

We've got to start somewhere, so let me begin by asking you a question. How old are you? Now, I know it's not the sort of question a gentleman asks. Nevertheless, I have a reason for wanting to know. Just to encourage you, let me confess: I am coming up to 50 years old. I was born in June 1946.

In the year I was born, ENIAC was also born. Who is ENIAC? ENIAC was the child of the University of Pennsylvania and is an acronym for electronic numerical integrator and computer. A newspaper clipping of the day reported:

IBM introduces fast electronic calculator

An 'electronic brain', capable of doing in seconds calculations that could take a human mathematician hours, is operating at the University of Pennsylvania. Known as ENIAC, the machine has 18 000 electronic valves, but no moving parts.

ENIAC is more than an electronic adding machine. It is a memory and can be 'programed' to do many different kinds of calculations. In fact, machines like ENIAC are bound to become major assets for scientists and engineers with complex and repetitive calculations to perform. They could find a role in commerce too, for processing things like pay-rolls.

Professor Douglas Hartree of Cambridge University, who played a part in the machine's evolution commented: 'The idea originated to assist gunnery in the war.' It is still in its infancy. The multiplicity of the problems which it can handle has not been defined.

Amazingly, this piece of news didn't make the front page of the papers. While I was researching I found it buried on the inside pages. It should have had front page banner headlines. It was thrilling, exciting, vital and would certainly make the earth move – it was the birth of the computer. At the time, no one understood the significance of what they were writing about, and I guess the truth is that Doug Hartree didn't know either.

Nineteen-forty-six was a vintage year. And I don't say that just because that was when I was born. No, it was a vintage year because events pointed the way to a new world. Some really good stuff was going on, getting started and about to happen. Some change levers were being pulled, new bells being rung, and the whistle was being blown to start a new game.

In 1946, newspaper readers will have noted that test flights had started to take place from a new, major airport to the west of London called Heathrow. The first plane to take off was from British South American Airways and was bound for Montevideo. Where's that?

And so it is, my lifetime has witnessed the birth of the computer, the introduction of the Biro, and the beginnings of Heathrow.

> '...we now spend 17.1 hours a week watching TV, half an hour a week in front of a computer terminal playing games, and millions of us jumped on an aeroplane to reach a holiday destination abroad'

I have also witnessed the development of computers into every nook and cranny of our lives: helping to put men on the moon and bring them home safely; playing a major role in conducting life-giving operations; and by the close of the century, the majority of homes will have access to some form of computing, predictions tell me. Ninety-six per cent of homes have a colour TV, but today only 2% of us have a TV of the sort conceived by John Logie Baird, with a black and white picture (*Social Trends*, 1995, HMSO, London).

If we are average (and no one I know will admit to that), we now spend 17.1 hours a week watching TV, half an hour a week in front of a computer terminal playing games, and millions of us jumped on an aeroplane to reach a holiday destination abroad.

I wonder what happened to British South American Airways? In just 50 years, a handful of inventions have changed our lives, and in my lifetime I expect to see the Biro become all but redundant as 'tablet screen' computer technology develops along with handwriting recognition software, and our computers learn to recognize both our voices and our scribblings.

All this in one man's lifetime

So, let me ask you the question again. When were you born? If you were born in 1951 you would have shared your birthday with the H-bomb. Who knows, you may also witness the redundancy of nuclear weapons. If 1960 is your birth year, a little chimpanzee called Ham is important to you. He was America's first space chimp, who splashed down safely, after his historic flight and was taken to Cape Canaveral – now called something else! Since which the US space programme has yielded thousands of viable new products.

'There is a centrifuge of technological advancement and change that, as it gathers speed, creates its own G-force and distorts the way we live'

The year 1970 saw the first jumbo jet land at Heathrow, and in 1971 pounds, shillings and pence gave way to decimal currency in the UK.

A fascinating game is to look back over your lifetime and chart the development of products and services and how they have changed what we do and how we live now. And then consider just how many of them we take for granted.

There is a centrifuge of technological advancement and change that, as it gathers speed, creates its own G-force and distorts the way we live. It was as recent as 1985 that the first person in the UK died of acquired immune deficiency syndrome (AIDS), as a result of receiving a transfusion of infected blood. Who knows where that hidden assassin will lead us unless medical technology kills it first? But as a result of it, our whole approach to the management of blood transfusion and donors has changed, and many young people in particular regard their sexual activities very differently from how we did 20 years ago.

Only ten years ago, a 15-day-old baby was given a baboon's heart and Clive Sinclair invented the electronic C5 tricycle. Promising so much, neither event has actually added much to our future. Animal-based alternatives to human organ transplants and man-made prostheses are still in the early stages of development and battery-powered vehicles still await the leap forward in technology that will eventually revolutionize travel.

It is worth remembering that it was the worldwide tidal wave of electronic computer-driven trading on the world's stock markets that, on 19 October 1987, fuelled a crash that wiped £50 billion pounds (10%) off the value of the London stock market, plunging thousands into terminal debt. This is yet another example of technology changing the way we live.

Permanent white water

I have an uneasy feeling about the future. The pace of history has speeded up. I am no longer sure we are masters of our future. A future driven by advances in technology makes what comes next unpredictable. It's exciting, I love it, but it worries me. I think we are facing a future driven by technology that will challenge our values, our beliefs and our institutions.

Let me give you an example: the Internet. It's wonderful, I love it, I play on it for hours, send messages, gossip, learn. I admit I am a greying old dodderer, but I am a born-again computer junkie. I mainline on the 'superhighway' that the Internet provides us with. It is a highway to fun, learning and communication, but it also poses questions that will challenge one of the foundations of modern society – the legal system. We will have to change our concepts of law, fairness and justice. Radical stuff.

'We will have to change our concepts of law, fairness and justice'

Why so? The Internet, an invisible web that currently connects about 40 million computer users with each other and news and information services on a global basis, is impossible to monitor. The astonishing number of people worldwide who are connected to the Internet, leaving a staggering number of messages and drawing off an incomprehensible amount of data, raises major concerns about the enforcement of copyright and pornography laws. Transactions can be too fast and too great in terms of volume for us to be able to police or exercise any meaningful control over them.

The kids are all into it in a big way. Homework and projects used to be a Biro drudge. Now, for an increasing number of kids, they are an electronic drudge. Need information for a project? Need to get some research done. Forget the library, burn the books (not this one, please!), get on the superhighway, access the forums, interrogate the directories and pull on to the screen just what the teacher ordered. Download it, place it on the homework page and print it out. Everyone is a genius.

Wait! Stop! Let's think about this!

Hold on a minute. So a student scans the Internet for data to complete a project. The student accesses an archive and downloads a drawing or photograph. How will the originator of the work receive a royalty for the use of it? The simple act of downloading data should initiate an audit trail that takes into account: authentication that the work of art is copyright to the person claiming to be the originator; a billing system for the person accessing the data; a payment system for the artist and for the banks to be able to track the transaction, on-line.

'We are likely to be driven to the role of spectator as copyright is consigned to history, or originators refuse to share their work'

Such a simple transaction will require an electronic banking system that is robust, error-free and can produce statements on demand. It sounds simple, but the computer architecture does not currently exist to support such transactions. Multiply that by one hundred million, the estimated number of electronic transactions that could take place in a year, and you see the size of the problem. There is no way the infrastructure, computer hardware and systems' architecture can be in place before the demand for them has come and gone, the damage done, the world moved on and in a real mess.

OK, so how will we enforce copyright law? Will we, in fact, be able to? Within the current processes of law, we seem to struggle to keep up with the simple demands of today, never mind the complex requirements of tomorrow.

We are likely to be driven to the role of spectator as copyright is consigned to history, or originators refuse to share their work. In which case, all incentive is lost. The very purpose of creativity disappears.

It gets worse!

Change the scenario. Let's make the work of art pornographic. The problems multiply a million-fold. Speaking at the 1995 Conference on Computers, Freedom and Privacy in San Francisco, Kent Walker, the district attorney who led the successful hunt for Kevin Mitnick, the world's most wanted hacker, said:

> When people are free to behave in anonymous ways, you will see a rise in antisocial behaviour. Anonymity is the urbanization of cyberspace.

I don't know what all that means, but it sounds bad to me!

Kent Walker had more bad news: 'strong encryption' (a way of securing data sent over the Internet), would make money laundering and tax evasion easier. He pointed out that a kidnap ransom paid in encrypted numbers, computer to computer, passed down 'phone lines, would be untraceable. Thanks Kent – nice thought!

The Governance of Cyberspace Conference at Teesside University in 1995 was told by Mike Whine, of the Board of Deputies of British Jews, that the

Internet was giving extremists 'unprecedented opportunities' for spreading racist and anti-Semitic propaganda.

The Internet provides access to services and sources that go beyond the law.

The Department of Health (DoH) is unable to prevent the sale of an illegal do-it-yourself testing kit for the human immunodeficiency virus (HIV, the virus that causes AIDS) that is being marketed on the Internet. The saliva-based test, developed in South Africa, boasts an accurate diagnosis in seven minutes. The DoH says it is unreliable and could lead people to attempt or commit suicide. DIY tests were made illegal in 1992, but because the Internet is beyond the powers of most UK laws, there is nothing the government can do. Ten saliva cards cost US $100 (about £64), mail order.

> 'We will be forced to compromise and reassess what we think'

Don't wait for the papers

The conference organizer, Dr Brian Loader, a senior lecturer in political studies at the university, said that Internet users had been able to read transcripts of the committal proceedings against Rosemary West, charged with 10 murders, which newspapers could not publish under the contempt of court rules.

So why wait for the papers? In fact, why wait for them anyway? I've always thought it strange that a multimillion pound industry depended on little boys and girls getting out of bed at some horrible time in the morning. Well, it looks like they can have a lie-in. Superhighway types can tap in:

http://www.telegraph.co.uk/.

and download a selection of material from the Daily Telegraph off the screen, just in time for breakfast. The paperboys and girls can still be dreaming of Nintendo. The rest of the papers will be on-line within 18 months, I bet! We used to wrap our chips in the papers, now the silicon chip delivers them.

The Internet, like so much new technology, will make us change our attitude to what is acceptable and what is not. We will be forced to compromise and reassess what we think. How we run our businesses and lead our lives will change radically, beyond the comprehension and reach of many of us. It was left to Dave Carter of Manchester City Council to make the final chilling point at the conference:

> **Within a few years, communicating via the Internet will be as familiar as using the telephone, but only if you have the necessary skills and can afford the technology in the first place.**

What happens to those who can't?

CHAPTER TWO

I know 'cos I was there

Thus I live in the world rather as a spectator of mankind than as one of the species
Joseph Addison

Some years ago I had the opportunity to travel, as a guest of the Konrad Adenauer Foundation, on a fact-finding visit to East and West Germany. The party comprised journalists, Members of Parliament and researchers.

I was dazzled by the affluence of West Berlin. I recall standing, dazed, looking into the windows of an ordinary West Berlin department store. Even for someone used to the delights and temptations of London's Knightsbridge, it was a shock. The quality, design and sheer elegance of the merchandise on display surpassed anything at home in London.

'Graffiti and symbols of remembrance; kisses and crosses side by side'

At that time West Berlin was a show case for West German industrial and economic success. West Berlin was a show-off city, and why not?

In contrast, East Berlin was almost indescribable. Grey, dull, uninspiring. Holes in the road, women queuing for black cricket balls that passed for cauliflowers. And then there was the wall. High, very high; higher than a house; enigmatic.

One section of the wall, near the Reichstag, was covered in graffiti. 'Flower power' drawings and messages of peace and love. Next to it, on a simple wire fence, hung several white crosses and a posy of flowers. They were suspended there in memory of the citizens who had lost their lives trying to climb the wall; swim the canal or tunnel under the land-mines; all of them willing to die in an attempt to escape to the West, rather than live in the East. Graffiti and symbols of remembrance; kisses and crosses side by side.

On the final evening of our trip we were the guests of the CDU, the German equivalent of the Conservative party. Its members told us of their manifesto commitment to reunite their country, 'one Germany'.

The next day, on the plane back to London, we reflected on the trip: the briefings we had had from the Bundesbank; the insights we had been privileged to be given; the UK ambassador; the lecture from the military chiefs of staff; and the conversations with the border police. To all of them and us, reunification seemed just a dream. We toasted the CDU in champagne and wished them well. Secretly, more than one of us laughed at their naïvety.

'I flew to Berlin and impounded my own piece of the wall to keep as a monument to my own short-sightedness'

Within three years of that visit the wall had vanished. On 9 November 1989 the old world moved into the future. The wall was not demolished by heavyweight politicians; it was pushed over by the citizens who had simply had enough.

No one had predicted the fall of the wall. It took the world by surprise. I flew to Berlin and impounded my own piece of the wall to keep as a monument to my own short-sightedness. The streets were heaving with people. The Westerners wearing designer jeans, the Easterners wearing disbelief. We drank beer, sang songs and slept on the street.

I have been back to Berlin again since, and all trace of the wall is gone. It is as though the past does not exist. The lesson is clear: expect the unexpected; planning is impossible, the pace of change too quick. It is the rate of change, the sheer speed with which events and developments take place, that makes conventional thinking redundant and ordinary reasoning superfluous.

Trapped in conventional thinking, some
organizations live behind a wall of their own
making, as prisoners of their corporate past. The
web of technological change is spun, not by
improvements whipped up at home, but by
international research and development over
which we can exercise no control or restraint.
Only one thing is certain: if you can imagine it, it
will happen; if you can't imagine it, you're out of it.

**'So turn the
page and look
back over
your own life'**

So turn the page and look back over your own life (Table 1). Have
a look for the turning points in history, that have taken place in your
lifetime, that have changed what we do, how we do it and what we
think.

Astonishing isn't it, how times have changed? The obvious turning points,
such as wars, are mentioned briefly on the list because the dates will be
indelibly etched on the minds of those who took part and in the
memories of those whose loved ones never returned – they need no
reminder. But, it is astounding to think that the first kidney transplant took
place in 1950, the contraceptive pill became available in the UK in 1960
and the first Jumbo jet landed in Heathrow in 1970.

Why stop at 1980? Firstly, because I didn't think anyone under fifteen
would be reading the book! But more seriously, because the pace of
change is almost too swift to record. Example? On today's calculations,
laptop computing power becomes 1000 times more powerful every ten
years! So, we have gone from the first giant computer-cum-adding machine
– ENIAC – demonstrated by Professor Hartree in 1946, through the
twilight years of the mainframe computer to the desktop box, and now, in
the last few years, to the palmtop replacement that is many times more
powerful.

Speaking at Nottingham University, in June 1995, BT's Head of Advanced
Applications, Professor Peter Cochrane, told a slightly stunned audience
that, by the year 2015, computing power will overtake the capacity of the
human brain.

Table I How has your world moved on?

1900 Trade unions create the Labour Party

1901 Daimler builds the first Mercedes car
Sweden awards the first Nobel Peace prize

1902 Thousands hit by smallpox outbreak
Discovery that yellow fever is carried by mosquitoes
Schools taken over by local councils
A trip to the moon is the first ever special effects movie, and is denounced as fanciful

1903 Royal Commission into London's traffic problems
Porcelain replaces gold fillings in teeth
Henry Ford founds motor company
First cataract operation
First flight by Wright Brothers

1904 Mr Rolls and Mr Royce make their first car
25% increase in the use of the postcard
Fingerprints first used in evidence in court case
Valves replace crystals in wireless sets

1905 Frenchman Alfred Binet invents the intelligence test
Einstein announces his theory of relativity
Aspirin goes on sale for the first time
London County Council's first ambulances introduced

1906 Britain's biggest battleship, the Dreadnought, built in four months
British Empire occupies one-fifth of the land surface of the globe

1907 Bill to build Channel Tunnel thrown out of Commons
British Medical Association (BMA) attacks evils of smoking
Lucitania crosses Atlantic in four days, 19 hours and 52 minutes
Vertical take-off first demonstrated in a French plane

1908 Edison patents motion picture projector
First open heart surgery, at St Joseph's Hospital, New York

1909 Blériot flies English Channel
House of Lords rejects 'People's Budget' to pay for poor

1910 X-rays guide removal of a nail from a lung
First Hollywood movie
Radio link captures murderer Dr Crippen at sea
Drug for the treatment of syphilis is the 606th to be patented
Florence Nightingale dies
Cancer thought to be caused by a virus

1911 1900 to 1911 UK population increases from 41.8 to 45 million
National insurance scheme unveiled
19 per 1000 die in British heat wave, mostly children
First airmail from Hendon to Windsor
Madame Curie wins Nobel prize for work on radium

1912 Titanic sinks
Nitrous oxide identified as safe anaesthetic
BMA fights National Insurance Act

1913 First moving assembly line at Fords
One in 100 children have ringworm or tuberculosis

1914 Start of First World War
British Empire has 1 million men under arms
Income tax doubled to pay for war
First 'bombs' thrown from aircraft

1915 Arms production slowed by drunken workers
Stonehenge sold for £6000 to Mr C H Chubb
Women factory workers twice as good as men

1916 Ford announces $250 touring car
Invention of tank to change the face of warfare
Loaf of bread costs 10d

1917 First aeroplane bombing of London

1918 Labour plans state control of industry
School leaving age raised to 14 years
Howitzer shells Paris from 65 miles away
Book by Marie Stopes (birth control pioneer) called Married Love discusses 'sex' and causes storm
10 million thought to have died in 'Great War'
Women vote for first time

1919 Rutherford splits atom
First air service links London to Paris
Alcock and Brown fly Atlantic non-stop

1920 Prohibition begins in the USA
Nellie Melba makes first advertised wireless broadcast

1921 First helicopter take off
First birth control clinic opened in London by Marie Stopes
7.4 million people live in London
Discovery of insulin gives diabetics hope

1922 Bohr wins Nobel prize for identifying structure of atom
First regular news broadcast
Inventor of X-rays (1895) Roentgen dies
Commission urges sex education to be taught in schools

1923 First transatlantic wireless broadcast made from UK to USA
First US astronaut Alan Shepard is born

1924 First Labour government
The UK's first national airline, Imperial Airways, takes off
First wireless conversation with Australia
Eight people die in UK's worst air crash, Imperial Airways

1925 British Optical Association denounces crosswords as the cause of eyestrain and headaches
US State of Tennessee makes it a crime to teach children the theory of evolution
Electric washing and wringing machine launched
First three-engine plane starts flying
Surgeon, Mr Souttar, dilated a faulty heart valve in a young girl. After exposing the heart he stretched the valve by poking his finger into it

1926 John Logie Baird demonstrates television
First rocket powered by liquid oxygen and gasoline launched in Massachusetts
General Strike

Airship flies over North Pole
Alan Chobham flies 28 000 mile
round trip to Australia

1927 February: Malcolm Campbell sets
world land speed record: 174.224
mph
March: Segrave snatches same
record at 203.841 mph, Daytona
Beach, Florida
Mae West jailed for lewd
Broadway show, Sex
Lindbergh makes first non-stop solo
transatlantic flight
1 729 000 motor vehicles on the
road in the UK

1928 £1 and 10 shilling notes
introduced. Labour objected saying
it would cause a recession
Amelia Earhart first woman to fly
Atlantic
UK has highest cigarette
consumption at 3.4 lb per head
Andy Warhol born
Professor Alexander Fleming
discovers Penicillium notatum

1929 1.6 million phones in the UK, 3.6
per 100 people
US Army plane flies 150 hours
non-stop
Segrave does it again! 231 mph
land speed record
Bentleys win Le Mans

1930 UK unemployment tops 1.5 million
TransWorld Airlines (TWA) formed
Since 1920, 250 000 new
buildings gone up in London
R101 airship explodes in ball of
flame
Wallace Carrothers discovers
nylon

1931 Aga cooker the centrepiece in
thousands of rural kitchens

Movies allowed to be shown on
Sunday for the first time
Empire State Building opened
First trolley buses run in London
Bentley Motors calls in the receiver
Thomas Edison, inventor of the
light bulb, stock-ticker machine,
and patentee of 1100 inventions
dies, aged 84

1932 Mersey Tunnel dug
Cambridge uses an 'atom
smashing machine'
Bell laboratories in the USA
discover radio waves from
constellation Sagittarius
German doctor Gerhard Domagk
discovers prontosil protects mice
against streptococci

1933 Hoover carpet cleaners on sale in
the UK for £4/19/6d
Oxford English Dictionary
includes new words: graft, once-
over, dope, step-on-the-gas, robot,
slimming, profiteer and Photostat

1934 274 000 new telephone
installations and 637 000 overseas
calls
Slimming craze blamed for the
slump in potato sales
In the previous 10 years
1 900 000 houses built in the UK
General Post Office (GPO)
introduces 'postal numbers' for
each district

1935 30 mph speed limit on roads
introduced
Royal Air Force (RAF) set to treble
in two years
Malcolm Campbell smashes 300
mph barrier in Bluebird
SS Jaguar, 90 mph touring saloon
launched at Motor Show

Robert Watson-Watt patents early radar device

Vitamin E obtained in pure form

1936 Volkswagen car launched
Spitfire I goes on show
Queen Mary on maiden voyage
BBC adds sound to TV pictures
Train ferry service from Dover to Dunkirk launched
Crystal Palace burned down

1937 Ark Royal launched
Hindenburg explodes

1938 First feature length cartoon – Disney's Snow White
Comic strip Superman launched
'Suburban neurosis' among housewives with nothing to do all day identified by doctor at Barnet Coroner's hearing
Mallard, a British train, tops 126 mph
80 000 ton Queen Elizabeth launched

1939 German physicist Otto Hahn discovers how to exploit energy in atom by the process of fission
Start of Second World War
Government plans to reclaim 1.5 million acres of derelict land for agriculture

1940 Queen Elizabeth on maiden voyage
Postage goes up to 2½d
Evacuation of British army from Dunkirk
Battle of Britain

1941 Pearl Harbor

1942 Monty triumphs at El Alamein
Beveridge Report heralds the beginning of the welfare state

1943 John Maynard Keynes 'invents' economic theories, including

International Monetary Fund

1944 Oswald T Avery discovers DNA
The 'prefab' house is launched
D-Day

1945 Potsdam conference shapes Europe of the future
A-bomb dropped on two Japanese cities
55 million dead during war

1946 IBM introduces first electronic calculator
First test flight from Heathrow
BMA launches £1 million fighting fund to defeat prospect of NHS
50 000 service divorces outstanding, 40% of girls are pregnant on their wedding day

1947 National Coal Board founded (nationalization)
Marriage Guidance Council gets government funding
Henry Ford dies
Reports that Russia is testing an A-bomb

1948 Medical consultants vote 766 to 11 to boycott the new NHS
Birth rate highest for 26 years
Infant mortality 41 per 1000, still births 24 per 1000
2751 hospitals form the NHS
Transistors replace valves in wirelesses

1949 45 rpm records launched
Comet jet airliner flies at 500 mph
Pound sterling devalued by 30%
10 times more divorces than in 1937
Convictions for drunkenness only half of pre-war rates

1950 Discovery of berkelium, the 93rd element
Robert Schuman, the French

Foreign Minister proposes a
Federation for Europe
US surgeon performs first kidney
transplant
First overseas TV broadcast by
BBC

1951 First H-bomb tested
Survey shows average housewife
works 15-hour week
90 mph hit of motor show

1952 Austerity forces government to
introduce NHS charges
One household in three lacks a bath
One in 20 has no piped water
First scheduled jet airliner

1953 Cargo doors on ferry left open, it
sinks off Belfast Lough
Successful test for polio vaccine
Stiletto heels denounced as
dangerous
Commercial TV to go ahead
Doctors to prescribe 'smog' masks
on the NHS

1954 Third British Overseas Airways
Corporation (BOAC) Comet
crashes, government grounds
planes·
Study finds cancer is linked to
smoking
IBM launches 'electronic brain' for
business use
Myxomatosis set to wipe out
rabbit population

1955 Motorway network planned for the
UK
Einstein dies, 18 April, aged 76
Campbell breaks water speed
record – 202.32 mph, Ullswater
First ITV broadcast
£40 British moped launched

1956 Self-service shops gets a mixed
reaction

Traffic wardens proposed
Suez

1957 Bank rate cut to 5%
Government refuses to ban
smoking
Macmillan says: '...most of our
people have never had it so good'
Sputnik 1, first in space
Contaminated milk from Windscale
poured down the drain
Laika, first dog in space, Russian

1958 USA puts first satellite into space
Hovercraft demonstrated
Parking meters in Mayfair, London
Bubble cars, £300 each
Ministry of Health warns about the
use of tranquillizers
Thalidomide first suspected of
causing birth defects
24.5 million TVs in UK, two-thirds
of adults own a TV, 34% view
BBC, 66% ITV
Filter-tipped cigarettes on sale
NASA picks astronaut squad

1959 Soviet rocket hits the moon
Lords oppose introduction of
commercial radio
M1 opened, police say design is
unsatisfactory
£20 million promised for new
London hospitals

1960 Britain to fund supersonic
aeroplane
Women with bare arms or dressed
as men to be denied the
sacraments by Catholic Church
Jodrell Bank sets space tracking
record of 407 000 miles
First 'weather lab' put into space
Jaguar takes over Daimler
Laser lighting first demonstrated

1961 Contraceptive pill goes on sale in UK

First American chimp in space
UK applies to join Common
Market
Soviet Union puts first man into
space
Berlin Wall built
1962 Smallpox outbreak
US astronaut is John Glenn
Stirling Moss crashes at 200 mph
Telstar launched
Cuban missile crisis
Polaris missiles to be used in
British submarines
Nelson Mandela first jailed, for five
years
60 deaths from London smog
Quasars discovered
Leeds General Infirmary carries out
kidney transplant in secret
1963 First metal tennis racket
Rachman housing scandal
Nuclear weapons test ban treaty
Hot line joins Washington with
Moscow
American Express launched in UK
Kennedy shot dead in Dallas
1964 Pirate radio starts
11-inch portable TV sold for first
time
USA and Russia launch Mars
space probes
Cigarette ads banned from TV
First US space walk
Church-going falls by 14%
TV watching up by 49%
1965 Mary Whitehouse launches 'clean-
up TV' campaign
Post Office Tower (620 feet high)
opened
First space docking by USA
Unmanned spaceship lands on
moon

1966 Harrier, world's first vertical take-
off plane, revealed at Farnborough
air show
Brain drain as UK scientists go to
the USA
British Motor Corporation strike
closes all car plants
1967 Flash fire on launch pad kills US
astronauts
Campbell dies as Bluebird
somersaults at 300 mph
Israel–Egypt Six Day War
Abortions to be legal in UK
Breathalyser introduced
World's first heart transplant, South
Africa
1968 First UK heart transplant
Catholics denied birth control
Epidural promises painless
childbirth
First abortion clinic opens in
London
Astronauts orbit the moon
1969 First moves to decriminalize 'pot'
smoking
Human egg is made fertile in test
tube
Concorde flies
Queen Elizabeth II's maiden
voyage across Atlantic
First man sets foot on the moon
First quins born to fertility drug
mother
1970 First jumbo jet lands at Heathrow
Range Rover goes on sale for
£2000
1971 Decimal currency introduced in UK
Rolls Royce goes bankrupt
First heart and lung transplant
1972 Britain joins European Economic
Community (EEC)
Divorces soar after Reform Act

Pound sterling to float on money markets

Granada, Ford's first internationally-made car

1973 Watergate
US Skylab in orbit
London Broadcasting, commercial radio, launched in competition with BBC

1974 Flixborough chemical explosion
US biologists claim genetic engineering may soon be possible
Ozone layer discovered to be threatened by chloroflurocarbons

1975 Cabinet split over Common Market (EEC)
Radio operated bleepers, telling people they are wanted, go on sale
Britain says 'yes' to Common Market in referendum

British Leyland to be state-controlled
Norton Villiers goes broke

1976 Bankruptcies hit all-time high
US Viking spacecraft lands on Mars
Space shuttle makes maiden voyage

1977 574 die in jumbo jet crash, Canary Islands
'Social contract' dead as wages claims soar

1978 Balloon sets record Atlantic crossing
UK announces it will not join EEC's new monetary system

1979 Three Mile Island atomic leak, USA
DC10s grounded in wake of crash in Chicago

1980 Modern medicine eradicates smallpox

The developments in medical technology, computing and robotics deserve a book of their own. Fed up with bulky mobile telephone batteries? How about a mobile phone that is powered from the body heat it picks up whilst in your pocket! It can be done. In the last ten years the world has undergone an invisible revolution. There is a thin veneer of the familiar – underneath it is all new.

What's next is anybody's guess.

CHAPTER THREE **The way we do what we do**

Confound their politics,
Frustrate their knavish tricks
Henry Carey

Powerlessness corrupts absolutely.
Me!

I have an uneasy feeling. I've not been able to put it into words, it is just a feeling. A feeling that is something like 'inevitableness', or 'powerlessness'. I get the feeling we're just not ready. As I go forward into the future I look back and reflect on a world that I don't recognize as the one in front of me. It's been very difficult to articulate what I mean. And believe me, I seldom have trouble with words. I am a natural-born gossip. I'm a talker. But I just couldn't get the words right for this. And then, *Bingo!* I came across some words that summed up what had been churning around in my mind.

> **The strength is there, but it is being sapped by a combination of weaknesses
> – a thousand wounds we find difficult to heal. We have weakened ourselves
> in the way we practice our politics, manage our businesses, teach our
> children, succour our poor, care for our elders, save our money, protect our
> environment and run our government.**

These words come from the American TV commentator John Chancellor in his book about the American way of life, *Peril and Promise, a Commentary on America* (New York, 1990).

For me, they sum up the struggle I have had putting into words what has been just a gut feeling. Perhaps disenchantment is too strong a word, and certainly I don't feel gloomy about the future. Quite the opposite, I think it *should* be exciting.

I guess my problem is: I'm not sure just how convinced I am about the weight I can put behind one of the words in that sentence. It *should* be exciting. I know it should, but I'm not convinced. We are going to have to be much more honest with ourselves about what comes next and we need to be a good deal more frank about where we are now before we can progress. I am not sure we can base our tomorrows on the foundations of today.

John Chancellor's words have become very important to me and I think they will become vital to us all. I do not believe it is possible to run an organization in a vacuum. Whatever goes on in the world outside our organizations will effect how we do business, how our staff are trained and educated, what motivates them and how they work, how successful our organizations are, how we find out what our customers are really after when they buy whatever it is we are peddling or shove in front of them when they've got no choices.

> 'Who is going to argue with me and say that there is not an undeniable relationship between all the nooks and crannies of society that John Chancellor highlights'

Who is going to argue with me and say that there is not an undeniable relationship between all the nooks and crannies of society that John Chancellor highlights in his chilling paragraph. It is chilling, isn't it? It's scary.

The political environment influences everything we do. Unemployment is a stepping stone to disenchantment and poverty. According to the Chief Constable of Sussex, poverty is a step away from crime.

An ageing population puts pressures on the state to provide services it can no longer afford. The result: more disenchantment with politics. I don't like it, it worries me, and if we are to survive we need a real rethink.

The kids are there already

Have you read the opening pages of this book? The bit that says: 'Aim: to develop a knowledge and understanding of the environment within which business activity takes place and the way in which changes in that environment influence business behaviour.'

It really is an extract from the Information Technology and Business Studies GCSE syllabus for 14-year-olds.

Think about it – 14! When I was 14 I was worried about getting into the football team and out from behind the bike sheds before my form-master caught me with Amanda Browne (I wonder what she's doing these days?). What were you doing when you were 14? I bet you weren't too worried about *developing a knowledge and understanding of the environment within which business activity takes place, blah, blah, blah.*

I've got news for you, you're going to have to develop it now!

The way we practise our politics

Well, it works, doesn't it?
Lord Callaghan

In very recent times the Japanese have lost a prime minister, the Italian political scene is too Mickey Mouse to describe, the USA has been beset with one scandal after another, and in the UK in 1995, a committee of enquiry, chaired by Lord Nolan, was set up to look into standards in public life. All this has been great for the sale of newspapers and has kept the journalists busy. But is it the real issue?

A look into the history books makes interesting reading. Politics has always been a dirty game and

'The French seem to have learned, quicker than most of us that politicians are just ordinary people in disguise and we should expect nothing from them that we do not expect from ourselves'

politicians are always getting caught at doing something they shouldn't be. Watergate and Profumo and before that Italian Mafia scandals and salacious revelations about personal sexual behaviour among the English upper classes. But none of this really matters. The French seem to have learned, quicker than most of us that politicians are just ordinary people in disguise and we should expect nothing from them that we do not expect from ourselves.

Out of the mainstream and into the menagerie

What does matter is the increasing disenchantment that the public have with politicians and the political processes that govern us. If you want proof, need an example, have a look at the USA during its last presidential election.

If ever there was a political process that is removed from reality, it is the US presidential election. I spent a few days there during the last one as an observer. I can tell you, US elections and the spin doctors, public relations experts and media manipulators make Coca-Cola and Pepsi marketing men and women look like the organizers of a car boot sale. These guys are experts with a capital EX!

It was perhaps during that election that I saw a glimpse of what is to come wrapped in the dynamic figure of Ross Perrot. The American public, tired of what was traditionally on offer, latched on to Perrot, and therein lies a lesson. He had made a success of his life and his business and the American people thought he could make a success of their lives and their businesses, too.

He made an impact in a race he never should have run, where he was an outsider and on uncertain ground.

Perrot spoke a different language and the

'...he had made a success of his life and his business and the American people thought he could make a success of their lives and their businesses, too'

American people translated it into a new beginning for themselves and their families. The interesting thing is that even today, nearly three years after the election, Perrot is still a big name in US politics. I was in Washington the day President Clinton's Health Reform Bill was withdrawn. Who made the headlines? Who was asked for a view? Ross Perrot. Newspapers are always quoting him. There isn't a big issue that goes by without he has not pronounced on it. US citizens wanted a change and they wanted Perrot. I think they still do.

The UK political scene is quite different, run at a different pace and with a structure that allows the razzmatazz and worst excesses of the US system to be avoided. But, look at the turn-out statistics for elections. In some elections for the European parliament the turn-out is less than 23%. Europe, with all the trouble that causes and three-quarters of us don't bother to have our say. Who cares what's going on?

A tiredness of politics. It is that tiredness that weakens us – one of John Chancellor's wounds.

The Henley Centre for Forecasting, one of the UK's leading think-tanks, called it, 'a sense of pervasive alienation from government and public institutions' in its 1995 'Frontiers' European research programme. It found that 64% of Britons were 'very or fairly' concerned about losing their job. They discovered that about 0.5 million professionals and managers in the UK were doing contract or temporary work. Gone is their dream of a job for life. Negative equity – the difference between the borrowing on a property and its market value – affects a quarter of all households in the UK.

People are in trouble, trying to dig themselves out of debt (Figure 1).

Bob Tyrrell, the Henley Centre's chairman, claims the underlying culprit responsible for our disenchantment, is global competition and its impact on employment. He thinks we may be driven to protectionism, which might preserve social cohesion but at the expense of a trade war, or to the creation of a new set of values emphasizing citizenship and altruism rather than the 'customer culture'.

'The underlying culprit ... global competition and its impact on employment'. I don't want to use the phrase 'global village' – it is just too much of a

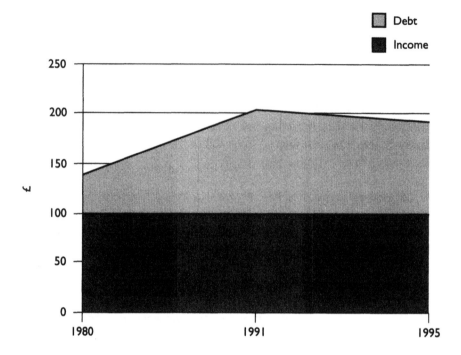

Figure I Debt to income ratio 1980–95 (estimate): personal debt for every £100 of income. (Source: 'Frontiers' European research programme, the Henley Centre for Forecasting.)

cliché. But how else can I describe it? Moving battle perhaps? When the fight arrives on your doorstep, who are your allies? Fight the fight, win, and the battle moves on; lose, and the battle moves on; perpetual, just-in-time battles.

David Walker, co-author of *The Times' Guide to the New British State*, writing in last summer's *RSA Journal*, said:

> One of the great political cries of our era is for greater accountability. There is a widespread public perception that a precious sense of public service is being lost from the administration of Britain, that disinterestedness is being replaced by cupidity and patronage. Quangos and the powers of government exercised through a menagerie of appointed bodies, have passed into the mainstream of party politics.

Today, more taxpayers' money is spent by unelected quangos than by local government.

Frustration with a political system that to some seems impenetrable and implacable is giving way to a new politics, a more dangerous politics. A 'New Age' politics.

Do-it-yourself politics

For years, the Campaign for Nuclear Disarmament (CND) marched its Easter march. Bruce Kent was there every year, and the annoying thing was he never seemed to get any older. The police earned a nice few quid in overtime payments, we all said, 'ooh' and 'aah' and not much changed.

Then came the environmental organization Greenpeace. We started to see what its members were up to on television – buccaneering things on the high seas and dangerous things with sewage pipes, interesting things with ropes, climbing high buildings, and embarrassing things when they ran rings around pot-bellied security guards. We stopped oohing and aahing and support them by giving money in street collections. They have uncovered dumps of chemicals and duplicity. They are pests and, in most cases, they are right.

> 'They have uncovered dumps of chemicals and duplicity. They are pests and, in most cases, they are right'

Then came the event that changed people's belief in the power of protest. The Poll Tax. The tax is cursed and has been the downfall of everyone who has tried it on. Over the years, the Poll Tax claimed the careers of cardinals and politicians and started riots. The scenes in Trafalgar Square must have told us something. Yes, I know some of them were thugs and opportunists, but many of the demonstrators in Berkshire and Surrey weren't.

Animal rights have gone full circle. Typified by the Animal Liberation Front, every bit the urban terrorists of protest, the headlines are now grabbed by elderly women chaining themselves to lorries at sea-ports. Tell me politics isn't changing.

Direct action. Motorway protesters are not all drawn from the great unwashed. Some are from the articulate middle classes and do not like what is happening to middle England. When the New Age traveller joins in common cause with the middle aged well-to-do, we know politics is changing.

> 'When the New Age traveller joins in common cause with the middle aged well-to-do, we know politics is changing'

People don't need the middle man any more. They don't have to trudge down to Westminster and lobby their MPs. They can let the world know what their beef is. People have got computers, they can wage war with a wordprocessor.

Motorway protesters perched in tree houses have mobile phones to talk live to radio stations. They have video cameras, and take their own pictures of the action to pass on to the TV companies in time for the evening news. They have fax machines, and bombard newsdesks worldwide with press releases.

Protesters are getting organized. They may not win all they protest about, but they don't half cause some grief for the authorities on the way. They have closed sea ports and closed businesses. They tie up resources to the point where some police forces don't have the money to put up a fight.

The new democracy doesn't need a ballot box. The new democracy is direct action. Democracy is protest. Guerrilla warfare, behind the lines attrition, clever, artful and highly organized protest.

Businesses find themselves with a new peril. Work in a business that turns out not to be politically correct and the protesters will close you down.

CHAPTER FOUR

Digging deeper

I like work: it fascinates me. I can sit and look at it for hours.
I love to keep it by me: the idea of getting rid of it nearly breaks my heart
Three Men in a Boat, Jerome K Jerome

Lack of vitality, confidence, call it what you will, in the UK's national institutions was nowhere better revealed than in a MORI survey of white collar workers carried out in the autumn of 1994.

Of those interviewed, 35% feared losing their jobs within the next year. Traditionally, white collar workers have been less susceptible to movements in the labour market. They are the last to experience redundancy and their managerial and administrative skills are highly transportable from one job to another. The survey dug deeper, and revealed that one in five families had experienced unemployment.

'These job losses are not just getting rid of the fat, they are structural. The job losses I'm talking about will change the make-up of the labour market for generations'

In most instances the cause of job loss is redundancy. Conventional redundancy is usually the consequence of 'de-layering' of the work force. So called de-layering is a euphemism constructed around the need to find another, more elegant way of saying: 'We're not doing the business and we've got too many people. So, goodbye'.

However, the job losses being experienced now are different. These job losses are not just getting rid of the fat, they are structural. The job losses I'm talking about will change the make-up of the labour market for generations.

Here is a copy of a slide I use when I am talking about **Futureproofing**. The slide deliberately has no title, and I ask the audience what they think the title should be. What title would you give it?

> **?**
> _____
>
> **British Telecom 100 000**
>
> **The banks 50 000**
>
> **Retail food stores 15 000**

The audience usually partly guesses the answer, they are half right. How about you? If you think the missing word is 'redundancies', you are half right too! Most people suggest that as the answer.

The correct answer is a more accurate definition of the type of redundancy. The correct answer is 'technology-based redundancies'. The fact is technology will rob more people of their jobs than recession ever will. Technology will take people out of the workplace and keep them out of it for a lifetime.

Unplugged

British Telecom (BT) is one of the great successes of modern technology and industry. Having shaken off the millstone of having once been a state-owned monopoly, BT is now truly a world-class company.

In my early days in business, getting connected to the telephone system was an art form. You almost had to know someone who worked in the Post Office before you could get the 'phone connected. Delays, heaped on waiting, followed by procrastination and the 'jobsworth' culture, made getting phones put in a new office a labour of love and frustration. Following the privatization of the telephone part of the Post Office and the birth of BT, restrictive practices have been swept aside and a new culture has appeared.

Have you called Directory Enquiries for assistance recently? No sooner is the number dialled than the operator replies. They are heart-attack fast. Does this new, fast, efficient service mean more jobs? Are there armies of operators waiting to pick up your call? No, there are fewer. The startling response times are the result of a computerized national call queuing system.

If you ring for assistance in tracking down a number from your desk in Brighton, the computer will connect you to the next available operator. Note the difference: *next available*, not the nearest. Geography is not the issue any more, availability is. For availability, read productivity. This means your request for a number could be answered in Manchester, Edinburgh or Birmingham. The system means fewer staff and a better service.

'Computer-based redundancies will never let people back into the workplace'

But that is not the end of the story. When the operator has answered your call and found your number, you are passed to a computer-generated voicebank that, in a Metal Mickey voice, tells you what you need to know. The system effectively halves the number of real people needed to run the service. Computer-based redundancies will never let people back into the workplace.

Banking on the future

It is the same story in the high street banks. More and more banking jobs will go – some predict 100 000 – as international electronic banking replaces people.

According to Sir Brian Pitman, chief executive at Lloyds Bank, about one-fifth of the existing industry workforce will disappear, on top of the 90 000 jobs that have already been lost over the past six years. The drive towards efficiency to combat intense competition and the increasing use of technology makes the banking sector, once one of the most secure white collar jobs, today one of the most insecure.

As Derek Wanless, chief executive of the high street bank NatWest, says:

> There is a huge amount of new technology to be brought to bear and that will remove a lot of traditional jobs. Anybody who pretends that is not the case is ignoring what technology can do.

I like that, the bit about '...anybody who pretends that is not the case is ignoring what technology can do'. We may not like the message but it is honest, direct, no messing. Derek Wanless isn't pretending.

Martin Taylor, the chief executive officer of Barclays Bank agrees.

> The banking industry will continue to lose thousands of workers every year. Clerical work of all sorts is clearly threatened.

Taylor goes further:

> ...the opening of European banking markets could bring a new round of rationalization. The European Union has close on 100 major retail banking institutions. There probably only need to be 20.

Shopping for jobs

Even the supermarket is a killing ground for computer-generated redundancy. This is probably a daft question, and I apologize, *everyone* goes to a supermarket but have you been to a supermarket lately? What a mess. Huge wide isles, canyons of consumerism, walls of good stuff to buy. Rush around or stroll, take your choice. Get to pay for the stuff and all hell breaks loose. Queues of trolley pushers waiting to pay. Can you imagine it. Waiting to pay! Actually waiting in a line to hand over their plastic or cash.

Tell that to a visiting Martian. Neanderthal! Well, I have news: within the next five years the congestion at the check-out will disappear, as will the check-out operator's job. Shoppers will add up the cost of what they have purchased on hand-held scanners and swipe their credit card to pay. The use of technology in the supermarket is long overdue. And that gets the prize for the biggest underestimate in this book!

Stores in The Netherlands, Scandinavia and the USA are already testing the do-it-yourself customer scanning system, and the scanners are currently being evaluated for use in the UK. Professor Gary Davies, of the International Centre for Retail Studies, has estimated that the technology could eventually cut retailing jobs by one-third.

> 'Professor Gary Davies, of the International Centre for Retail Studies, has estimated that: "... technology could eventually cut retailing jobs by one-third" '

In the Gledermaisen store of Albert Heijn, the largest Dutch supermarket chain, shoppers attach handheld scanners to their supermarket trolleys and electronically read the bar codes on the goods they've chosen. When shopping is complete, the scanner prints out the bill. Heijn claims the system, introduced in 1993, has increased sales and profits, because it has improved the accuracy of pricing.

Why is it still 'on trial' in the UK? What is going to be discovered that Albert Heijn doesn't know already? For goodness sake, go and buy the kit, install it in my local supermarket and let me get out of the queues!

There is more

In 1995, Tesco, one of the UK's leading food retailing outlets, has introduced a Customer Loyalty Card. The headline reason for the card is to reward loyal customers in a competitive market by giving them bonus points and discounts. Tell me the real reason is not to build up a picture of

> 'A greater craftiness is on the way and I love it'

what an individual customer buys, ready for the day when supermarkets deliver basic repeat-order products to your door, paid for by direct debit, straight out of your bank.

Then the high-cost, edge-of-town, capital intensive, costly to repair and maintain, floorspace could be halved. The next step will be for us to do the rest of our shopping on TV. Far fetched? Have a look at Channel 12 on BSkyB satellite TV.

CHAPTER FIVE

Unemployment

I'm going to work, and in twenty-five or thirty years' time every man and woman will be working
Three Sisters, Anton Chekhov

If what the Hudson Workforce 2000 Study (Hudson Institute, New York, 1994) tells us is true, there is an inextricable link between education and work.

How much of this did you know already?

- By the year 2000 more women will be working than men.

- *Two out of three women now work full-time.*

- There are about 127 000 males aged 18–24 who have been unemployed for a year or more.

- *Only 38 000 women fall into the same category.*

- Six months after leaving university, 45.4% of female graduates are in work, compared with 42.3% of male graduates.

- *After a year, 12% of male graduates are unemployed, compared with 8% of women.*

- The number of women entering management schools was around 10% a decade ago. It is now 20–30% and rising.

- *Researchers predict that within a decade teaching will be an all-female profession.*

- At school, boys lag behind girls in every subject.

- *In 1993, 45.8% of girls achieved five top grade GCSEs, compared with only 36% of boys.*

- Girls are twice as likely as boys to get a grade A in A-level English.

- Boys outnumber girls two to one in UK schools for children with learning difficulties.

- *In special units for children with behavioural problems, there are six boys for every girl.*

- 80% of girls plan to go on to college, compared with only 60% of boys.

- Young men represent one-eighth of the population, but commit one-third of all crimes.

- *The suicide rate among young men has risen by 70% in the past decade.*

- Young men (15–24) have a suicide rate of 16 per 100 000; *the rate for girls is five per 100 000.*

Fact or fiddle?

I keep worrying about technology knocking people out of the workplace and the government keeps telling me unemployment is going down. None of this makes any sense. Somebody must know what the situation is. Let's start by having a look at how the numbers are counted.

Two methods are used to count the number of unemployed. The claimant count and the labour force survey, both published by the Department of Employment.

The claimant count

This count is taken from administrative statistics and comes out once a month. In most Western countries, unemployed people register at state offices either to look for a job, or to receive benefits, or both. In October 1982, UK job seekers were no longer required to register with Job Centres as well as with the Benefits Offices, and the count was switched to people claiming benefit.

First problem; not all unemployed people claim benefit and not all unemployed people are entitled to benefit. Although unemployment benefit is not means tested, you do have to have made enough National Insurance contributions, paid during previous employment, to qualify. If you are not eligible for benefit you don't appear in the count.

The introduction of the Job Seekers' Allowance in 1996, will have an impact on the claimant count that is yet to be assessed. Statisticians believe the allowance will have an effect on claimant behaviour and make the claimant count inconsistent.

The Labour Force Survey

The Labour Force Survey started in 1984, when it was annual; since 1992 the numbers have been published quarterly. A market research-based approach, it covers 60 000 households and captures data from about 120 000 people over 16 years of age. Each quarter, 20% of the households are changed and interviews are carried out, face to face at first, and subsequently by phone. The Survey covers unemployment, employment, self-employment, hours of work, redundancy, education and training.

Working or not or what?

- A friend has a son, bright lad, just left university as a science graduate. He's looking for a job. Saturday evenings he plays in a band, in a pub. He gets paid for that in cash. He is 21 years old. Is he employed or unemployed?

- My cousin's daughter lost her job when the factory she was working in closed down. The girl is 17 years old and works only for three hours on Saturday mornings packing shopping bags at the cash desk at the local supermarket – the only job she can find. Is she employed or unemployed?

- A neighbour runs a small graphic design business. His brother, aged 55 years, also a designer, is out of work and drops into the business to help out, just to keep his hand in and keep up with what is going on. My neighbour can't afford to pay his brother, but they usually end up in the pub on the way home. Is he employed or unemployed?

The answer to all three questions? Employed.

Who says so? The International Labour Organization at its 13th International Conference of Labour Statisticians in October 1982. So there!

Definition

Employment: All aged over 16 years who did some paid work (whether as employed or self-employed) during the counting period ... those working in a family business on an unpaid basis are identified within this group.

This is daft. You and I know the real definition. The only definition that is worth a carrot, and the only numbers worth counting, are found in the answers to the common-sense questions: 'Do you have a proper job?' and 'Would you like to have a proper job?'

Don't let's get bogged down in what a 'proper job' is. We know it is unlikely to be playing in a band, in a pub, once a week; packing shopping in a supermarket on Saturday mornings or slaving over a hot computer for the reward of a free pint on the way home.

Economists hang on to the figures because, to them, unemployment is a downward pressure on wages and hence inflation.

The sociologist sees the figures in a completely different light – how much labour is available and how the world of work meets the demand.

Table 2 shows the number of changes there have been in how we count the number of people out of work.

I'll leave you to total it up, but I would guess the changes have reduced the total of jobless people shown by the statistics by more than 1.3 million.

> 'The only definition that is worth a carrot, and the only numbers worth counting, are found in the answer to the common-sense questions: "Do you have a proper job?" and "Would you like to have a proper job?"'

Table 2 Changes in how the number of people out of work are counted*

Change	Year of change	Impact on jobless figures (+/−)
Benefits paid fortnightly	1979	+20 000
Downward adjustment of seasonal total		−20 000
Estimated effect of first training schemes	1981	−19 555
Adjust for strike at DHSS†		−20 000
Men aged 60+ no longer required to sign on		−30 000
Only benefit claims counted	1982	−216 000
Men aged 60+ not required to register for NI‡ credits	1983	−107 000
Men aged 60+ allowed long-term supplementary benefits		−54 000
School-leavers barred from benefits for one to three months		−200 000
Community programme rule change	1984	−29 000
Northern Ireland reconciles DHSS† records and files	1985	−500
Two-week delay introduced in announcing statistics	1986	−50 000
New method of calculating percentage of unemployment		−1.4%
Abolition of part rate unemployment benefit		−30 000
Voluntary unemployment disqualification extended to 13 weeks		−3000
Availability for work test toughened		−300 000
Voluntary unemployment disqualification extended to 26 weeks	1988	−12 000
Youths aged 16 and 17 years barred from benefits		−120 000
Unemployment benefit contributions tests toughened		−38 000
Some 55–60-year-olds switch to pensions instead of benefits		−30 000
Ex-miners not required to register	1989	−28 000
Claimants required to be looking for work		−25 000
Low wage levels no longer reason to refuse job		−25 000
Tightening of regulations to re-qualify for benefit		−350
Change to the way earnings affect right to benefit		−30 000

*Source: Royal Statistical Society, working party report, 1995.
† Department of Health and Social Security (as was).
‡ National Insurance.

There are two other definitions 'unemployed' and 'not looking for work'. Bring the three definitions 'employed', 'unemployed' and 'not looking for work', together in a fluid and flexible labour market and a unique and unexpected conundrum appears.

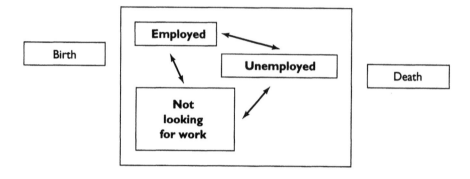

Figure 2 Turbulence in the labour market.

Look at the employment process. School-leavers look for work at different ages: they are 15 or 16 years old if they leave school early, 18 or so if they leave after A-levels, or in their early 20s if they carry on into further education. Within the labour market there is turbulence as workers move in and out of employment; having passed the age of retirement is no assurance that they will no longer look for and secure work.

Now let's explore the flowchart in Figure 2 in conjunction with the figures from the Labour Force Survey for women in the summer of 1994 (Table 3), and find out what it all really means.

Let's look on the bright side and imagine some jobs became available and 1% of women not looking for work were attracted back into a job. At the same time, the jobs attract 10% of the unemployed women. There would be 107 000 moving from 'not looking for work' to 'employed', and 90 000 moving from 'unemployed' to 'employed'.

Table 3 Labour Force Survey of women in the summer of 1994

| | Estimated number (millions) | | |
	Employed	Unemployed	Not looking for work
Female	11.3	0.9	10.7

Although a much bigger proportion moved from *unemployed* than from *not looking*, the impact of the new jobs on the size of the unemployed pool would be quite modest because of the much larger size of the *not looking* groups.

Here's the important bit. Because of the way we count the *unemployed*, fewer than half of the new jobs becoming available would show up in a reduction in the number of *unemployed*.

With apologies to Disraeli: there's lies, damned lies and government statistics!

You pays your money and you takes your choice

The claimant count is fast and comes out once a month, but it excludes a lot of people that common sense tells us are really unemployed. The Labour Force Survey is expensive to do and takes three months to get to us, and it may not be accurate by the time we study it.

The problem with unemployment figures is they have to be all things to all people. They are used by a variety of people:

- politicians who want to prove their policies are working
- economic policy-makers, finance institutions, trade unions, local authorities and business, who want to plan for the future
- social commentators and journalists, who have a variety of motives.

Neither of the two sets of statistics suits all parties and consequently no one believes them any more. Real achievements are overlooked and real problems go unspotted. What else could we do?

The Royal Statistical Society's Report of the Working Party on the *Measurement of Unemployment in the UK*, published in 1995, comes up with four brilliant ideas.

- A measurement attached to the labour force based on hours (so simple why didn't we think of it?).

- A measurement of long-term unemployment based on failure to find 'real work' (training courses don't count).

- A social measurement of the number wishing to work (they do it in The Netherlands).

- A separate measurement of the 'young' unemployed.

If we are to plan for the future we need real facts: numbers that stand up and statistics that tell us the truth. Part of preparing for the future is to be honest about where we are today. Statistics that are less than cold-steel-straight about where we are, fool us into a false sense of security and mislead our conclusions about what we must do next.

Have a go at answering the questions in Table 4 to see what you must do next.

Table 4 How will technology-driven redundancies influence you?

You

- *Is your job on the line? Are you techno-proof? If you think you are, buy 200 copies of this book, pile them high and jump off the top – you're out of it.*
- *Do you have up to date skills? How up to date? Are you still doing your job like you did it five years ago – you won't in the next five years.*
- *Can you get new skills? Of course you can – but don't take too long. By the time you have learned something it could be out of date.*
- *How will you assess what skills you need?*

Your organization

- *Can you stay competitive with the levels of technology you have now? Don't bother to think – the answer is no!*
- *Will you improve competitiveness with higher levels of technology? Or, is it just about survival?*
- *Can you afford the investment? Can you afford not to? Technology is cheap.*
- *What will it mean for staffing levels?*
- *Are redundancies manageable in public relations terms?*
- *What transition period are you likely to go through?*

Your market

- *Is your market technology driven? Of course it is – daft question.*
- *Do you have any control over the introduction of new technology? You might in your business, but step outside the door and the answer is no.*

Your suppliers

- *Will your suppliers survive? Some may go – get multisourced.*
- *Can you work with them in the introduction of technology such as electronic data inputting (EDI) links?*
- *What effect will it have on prices – up or down? Only down will do as an answer.*

Where do you fit?

Track your path from where you are to where you need to be. Score more than seven and you shouldn't be sleeping well at night.

Fast adjuster	1		1	Low-tec risk
		2		
Slow adjuster	5		4	High-tec risk

CHAPTER SIX

Trampled in the rush

La maison est une machine à habiter.

A house is a living-machine.
Le Corbusier

The 'march of technology' is a phrase we are all used to. You read it in the papers, hear about it on the telly, yeah, yeah, cliché stuff. But, it's true. It is horrifying.

Have a look at these figures and see what we have given birth to. In the final quarter of 1994 personal computer (PC) software sales in Europe rose by a staggering 11% to US$540.2 million. The UK is Europe's second largest software market, just behind Germany (Figure 3).

Software sales are not the only measure. Some argue they are misleading. They say as new software is developed, old systems become redundant. The figures include 'churning', the turnover of replacement software, people moving to a higher specification, upgrades and the like. OK, who am I to argue? Let's have a look at something else.

A very revealing figure is hardware sales. The number of people planting a PC on their desk. Few businesses can exist without computers, but they are also upgraded, so there is more churning.

Take a look at people who are most likely to be getting a PC for the first time. The domestic market. According to the GfK Market Research Services Report on the Sale of Electrical Equipment for the UK Domestic Market in 1994 (published 1995), British households spent more on computer equipment for the home than on any other consumer durable, more than on hi-fi, video recorders or even TVs (Figure 4).

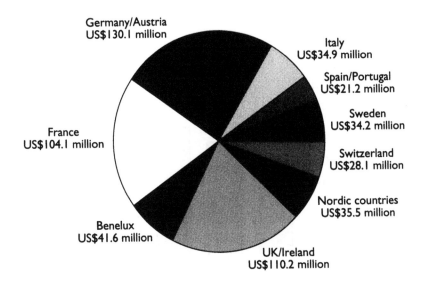

Figure 3 Personal computer software sales in Europe in 1994. (Source: *Wall Street Journal* analysis, 28 March 1995.)

None of this was junk, or toys for the kids. No, this was high specification, high quality equipment. Well over half the purchases included a CD-ROM drive. The average price of a computer was just over £1000.

Sales of PCs have soared by 55% in the UK. Research by Wharton Information Systems shows sales zoomed to £3.1 billion, an increase of 55% on 1993. Hardware manufacturers spent £67 million on advertising, with £14 million spent in December 1993 alone.

Rice Homes, a property development company, and Compaq, the PC manufacturers, are joining forces to build the UK's first 'computer friendly home' in Ashford in Kent. The homes will have pre-installed networks, featuring data sockets in

'According to Lloyds Bank Small Business Unit in 1995, more than two-thirds of small businesses admit they are having trouble keeping up with changes in information technology'

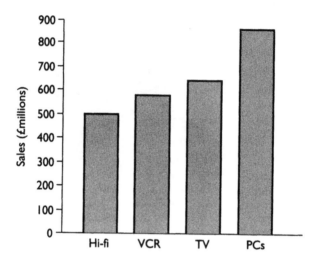

Figure 4 Sales of electrical equipment in the UK domestic market in 1994. (Source: GfK Marketing.)

every room, three telephone lines for fax, modem and access to the information superhighway. Buyers of the homes will also get an information technology service from Compaq dealers offering them advice, installation and training packages to help with home computing!

The PCs going into peoples homes are not just going to sit on a desk and be decorative. The purchase of computers at this level will have a major impact on the capacity for home working, home shopping and home education – times are a-changing! But what into?

CHAPTER SEVEN

What's it like over at your place?

And make the babbling gossip of the air...
Twelfth Night, Shakespeare

The organization is a concept and is nothing more than an address.

The relationship between knowledge workers and their organization is a distinctly new phenomenon.
Peter Drucker, *Harvard Business Review*

How would you like to open your postbag one morning and get a letter like this:

Dear Employer

I'm looking for a job. I have taken care to make sure my knowledge and skills are up to date. I am loyal, hard-working, presentable and full of energy.

I want to work in a place that will care about me as much as I will care about you. Somewhere that is profitable but not greedy and does things for the community I live in. Somewhere that is conscious of the fact that resources are finite and doesn't chuck anything nasty into the atmosphere.

Somewhere I can work through until three in the morning if I feel like it and somewhere I can have my pet goldfish on my desk. I want to have fun at work, opportunities to learn and develop as a person. I want a workspace that I can decorate to fit my own character and a window to open if I want.

Yours hopeful

Hands up if you'd throw the letter in the bin? Tell me I'm a crank, but I would quite like to get a letter like that. I would quite like to meet the person who wrote it. I would very much like to be able to say 'yes' to all the questions.

Getting the right people and keeping them is not easy. What we offer people and how we look after them goes beyond the conventional work station, a nine-to-five routine and a water fountain.

Offices are designed by people who do not work in them. Office space is allocated by people who work somewhere else. Desks are dished out on a 'departmental' basis. All one herd in one cage. One species in one enclosure. The finance corral, the personnel pen; all designed to encourage corporate tribalism, reinforcing just what we don't want reinforced!

> 'What we offer people and how we look after them goes beyond the conventional work station, a nine-to-five routine and a water fountain'

Organizations do not have to revolve around buildings, and increasingly they will not. The increasing use of technology, not just in the workplace but, more significantly, at home, is bringing us closer to the time when, as the organization gets bigger it can actually get smaller.

There are whole industries devoted to making sure we don't have to go to work. There are fortunes being made out of software, hardware and the latest (wait for it) floppyware, to make sure we are wired up, connected, linked and communicating wherever we are.

There's a copper at the front door

Until recently, British Telecom (BT) has been in something of a fix. The big question was how to get in on the act. There are very few buildings in this country that don't have a piece of BT wire running up to the front door. The problem for BT was that the wire is made of copper, which is slow to conduct data. Fibre-optic networks can perform much better. BT knows this and have wanted to use their fibre optic network – they have 3.5 million kilometres installed already.

You know how I feel about BT? It is a world-class outfit. It has been ruthless on jobs but it has had to be. BT is one of the UK's major success stories. However, the government, in its infinite wisdom and commitment to competition (ho, ho, ho), and in an effort to give the fibre-optics newcomers a head-start, has banned BT from delivering real time broadcast TV into fibre optics until the year 2001.

While the fibre-optic industry was counting its blessings, putting on its hard hat and starting to dig up every street in the UK, burying its cables, BT's research and development laboratories at Martlesham Heath in Ipswich put on their thinking caps and dug down to find a technological breakthrough. They have come up with a way of sending the equivalent of 60 A4 pages in just 30 seconds, compared with the more than 20 minutes it takes using a modem.

'... the whole thing is such good quality that one presenter for the radio station Classic FM broadcasts live from his home in the Cotswolds using the technique'

Called Integrated Services Digital Network (ISDN), it is able to exploit the whole frequency bandwidth of copper wire and works like using lots of modems in parallel, sending two megabits of data per second. BT claims it has better quality pictures than VHS.

Indeed, the whole thing is such good quality that one presenter for the radio station Classic FM broadcasts live from his home in the Cotswolds using the technique. What I am getting around to saying is that teleconferencing will soon be a 'plug-in and play' reality for every business and organization. The copper wire at your front door is a pathway, a trailblazer, a track and a scout that will take you anywhere. And it worries me!

Where do we put the water fountain?

If we sit at home doing our jobs, reporting in, talking to each other on a TV screen, sending data down the line, what will happen to management by huddle, who will make the water fountain decisions? I am very torn. Torn between what I think will happen and what I know we need to do to make things happen.

I cannot believe that technology will not play its part in breaking up the Jurassic Parks that are the buildings we constructed as temples to our ambitions. Buildings built with foundations in the past and no windows on the future. Of course they will go. They will go and release the huge tranches of capital tied up in heating, lighting and maintenance services. The impact this will have on capital values and balance sheet structures is something nobody wants to get to grips with. For many companies, the value of the buildings they occupy underpins much of their activity. Nowhere is this more true than in the National Health Service (NHS) where, in the past 10 years, average bed-stays have fallen from 10 days to 6.5 days; the throughput in UK hospitals has gone up by 30%. NHS hospitals are, at the very least, in the BT class for performance based on improvements in technology.

Yet still the NHS struggles to close its clapped out buildings as politicians, union leaders and the press whip up a public debate based on an attachment to historic buildings rather than on real reform that will lead to low cost, high quality services.

Up to 30% of an organization's overheads can be spent (or wasted) on heating, lighting and air-conditioning, and all the other headings that are dead money for a business. People leave their heated, well lit, comfortable homes behind and struggle to arrive at workplaces that are less comfortable but equally well lit. The temptation to ship the work to them instead of shipping them to work is overwhelming.

So, yes, I know all this and I want you to know I am not in the business of knocking it. But I am worried.

If we ask ourselves the question: 'What makes

'...in the NHS... in the past 10 years, average bed-stays have fallen from 10 days to 6.5 days; the throughput in UK hospitals has gone up by 30%. NHS hospitals are, at the very least, in the BT class for performance'

businesses work? What makes real success?', the answer has to be the people who work in it. Bill Gates, boss of Microsoft says:

> A company is only limited by the imagination of the people who work in it.

If every one is sitting at home chatting on the Internet, waving at each other through BT's ISDN, where does the inspiration come from? Where do we put the water fountain?

'What is the workplace if not a theatre? People on show, putting on a show, listening to the applause when it all goes right and the boos when it doesn't'

What is the workplace if not a theatre? People on show, putting on a show, listening to the applause when it all goes right and the boos when it doesn't. Define where people work as something other than a showring. They are in the ring performing, doing the tricks that earn them their living; hearing the cheers from the crowd, they are egged on to jump higher, run faster, score more points. Work is social. Work is interaction. Good work is fun. Think again about that letter in your post bag. Let's pull it apart and see what it really says.

I want to work in a place that:

- will care about me as much as I will care about you
- is profitable but does things for the community I live in
- is conscious of the fact that resources are finite and doesn't chuck anything nasty into the atmosphere
- I can work in through until three in the morning if I feel like it
- lets me have my pet goldfish on my desk
- I can have fun at, while working
- offers me opportunities to learn and develop as a person
- gives me a workspace I can decorate to fit my own character
- gives me a window to open if I want to.

Where is 'Hopeful' describing? The nearest place I can think of is *home*, and it is dangerous.

Home is where the couch potato grows

Home is comfortable but it is not creative. There is no gossip and gossip is at the heart of team-building, togetherness, close-knit and crew. What can we add to the list of theatre and showring? What else can where we work be? Home-from-home may not be a bad bet.

Creativity is not compartmental. Creativity is porous, it kind of leaks out. Creativity does not surface in formal surroundings. Go to Silicon Valley and talk your way into any of the software houses there and look around. You will find offices that look like playgrounds.

'Creativity is not compartmental. Creativity is porous, it kind of leaks out'

The parish pump is where the decisions used to be made. Bedouins collected around the wadi and old crones around the teapot. The water fountain is where the decisions are made, the ideas get swapped and water turns into a team spirit.

Nipping into someone's office for a chat about this or that, a few words exchanged in the car park in the morning, may all set the tone or idea for the day. Scheming, plotting, competing. All of these creative niches will be lost if we all work from home.

To **Futureproof** our organizations is to preserve gossip, protect niche communication and find a place for the water fountain.

So what do we do about keeping the team together? Easy. Turn your office into a club, a social centre, a meeting house, a night club, a society. Anything, make it a place people want to drop into. David Teasdale used to run the UK subsidiary of the German medical supplies group Fresenius. He lived on E-mail, faxes and voice-banks. Now he's moved on and opened his own company.

'What are your offices going to be like?' I asked him.

'Small, like a drop-in centre', he said.

And, what is more, he means it. Work where you are, at home, on a plane, on a train, in your customer's office but drop into the office for fun and gossip. Back to the studio to be creative. Back to the funny farm for the new ideas, vision and creativity. Bounce the ideas, get a reaction and react.

Have fun by the water fountain.

'Turn your office into a club, a social centre, a meeting house, a night club, a society . . . make it a place people want to drop into'

CHAPTER EIGHT **Get educated, get a job, er ...**

Human history becomes more and more a race between education and catastrophe.
H G Wells

I look back on my school days and cringe, I hated the experience and couldn't wait to get out. I'm maybe just old enough to get away with it. I am a lost cause. But, in an increasingly complex world it is not hard to understand the importance of education. The Hudson Institute's Workforce 2000 Study predicts that by the end of the century, 52% of new jobs will require a college education. Easy enough to understand. New jobs will require new skills, new skills will need new training.

> 'The Hudson Institute's Workforce 2000 Study predicts that by the end of the century, 52% of new jobs will require a college education'

The problem with all this is that two-thirds of UK workers currently have no vocational or professional qualifications. Today's standards of education, translated into the workplace, mean that, for example, at a UK car manufacturing plant seven out of 10 job applicants fail to score 40% in a verbal reasoning test.

In Germany they face different problems. A German engineering apprenticeship takes four years to complete. The problem is, that the half-life of the skills the apprentices acquire is also four years.

Put another way: most of what the German apprentices learn is out of date by the time they come to apply their knowledge. A graphic example of how technology overtakes education.

Tell me, when it takes 14 years to become a consultant in a UK NHS hospital, just how much knowledge has passed its 'use by' date by the time it is applied?

So, how are we doing? Are we all polished up and ready to go? You'd better take a look at Figure 5. If, as the Hudson study (see page 33) tells us, workplace qualifications are important for the future, we've got a problem.

According to an independent report by the Organization for Economic Co-operation and Development (Education at a Glance, International Comparisons, Paris, 1995), the UK spends 4.1% of its gross domestic product on education, ranking it

'...at a UK car manufacturing plant seven out of 10 job applicants failed to score 40% in a verbal reasoning test'

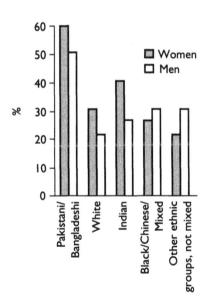

Figure 5 Percentage of working population without qualifications. (Source: Department of Employment, 1993.)

ninth out of 13 nations, including the USA, Ireland, Denmark, Finland, Portugal and Sweden. The report also shows that British classrooms are among the most crowded, with 15.1 pupils per teacher at secondary level, ranking it 12th out of the 18 countries listed. Does that figure of 15.1 pupils per teacher sound strange? It did to me, particularly with all the recent publicity about large class sizes. What's the explanation? Easy. Not all teachers are teaching at the same time! This is particularly true in secondary schools where teachers will have periods 'scheduled out' for marking, preparing lessons, etc. This is less true of primary schools where nearly all the teachers teach nearly all of the time. Nevertheless, take the number of pupils, divide by the number of teachers and this is what you get.

> '...by the time Japanese students are 14 years old, they have received as much education as their 17-year-old British counterparts'

You won't be surprised to learn that it's a bit different in Japan! The teacher–pupil ratio is about one teacher to 20 children. There is a rigid formality about Japanese schools. Each student receives nine years of compulsory education, with 90% of pupils continuing on to high school – a rate well above that in the UK or the USA.

The literacy rate in Japan is 93% and the number of days a Japanese student attends school per year is about 220, including Saturdays! In the USA the school year is roughly 180 days and in the UK it is about 165 days. It would be interesting to know which of these factors (if any – or perhaps it's all of them) result in an average Japanese student scoring 117 in a standard intelligence test while Europeans score 100.

Never short of free coffee

Back in my school days I remember there was a coffee bar on the way home. We were not allowed to go into the coffee bar – it was regarded by the school, parents and anyone over 35, as a den of iniquity. It had a juke box and a pin-ball machine. Like all forbidden places, it was irresistible, and when school was over a crowd of us would dive into it. The place was owned by a sinister and very volatile guy whom everyone assumed to be Greek, hence he became 'Nick the Greek' and the café became known as Nick's place.

Nick was a very good business man. Not only did he understand that forbidden fruit tastes the best (and so never complained about the fact that the school put his place out of bounds), but he also gave a week's free coffee to whomever made the week's highest score on the pin-ball machine. For school boys existing on what they could cadge from their parents or screw out of a miserly weekend employer, this was a prize worth playing for.

Winning on the machine was never easy. I remain convinced he fixed it. But such is the resourcefulness of youth that we discovered that if four of our largest rugby players stood at each corner of the machine and lifted it ever so slightly off the ground, we could tilt the playing surface and gently roll the ball into the 500 hole every time, all without the tilt light coming on and the bell ringing, alerting Nick to the fact we had cheated. Boy, did he get mad if he caught us!

We were never short of free coffee. The lesson I learned in Nick's place was more valuable than anything I learned at school: if you want to be sure to win, get things tilted in your direction. Education is about tilting the playing field in your direction.

Conventional education starts with school, progresses to college or university and then on into the workplace. Once there, the firm will provide training that is usually job-specific. The notion that the firm looks after the employee in a mutual pact is matriarchal. What is good for the one is usually good for the other. That is a level playing field (or pin-ball machine) and that is OK.

Or is it? What is good for one may not be so good for the other. Training that is job-specific

> **'The lesson I learned in Nick's place was more valuable than anything I learned at school: if you want to be sure to win, get things tilted in your direction. Education is about tilting the playing field in your direction'**

may not be transferable, and the employee may thus get trapped in a position that is difficult to break out of. This situation is compounded if the work comes to an end and the employee is made redundant. If the skills are job-specific, the employee is stuck. During the mid-1980s, to their cost the miners, train drivers and steel workers discovered this to be true. Add to this the complication that technological developments are making conventional work skills redundant, and the employee can be in a mess.

Note, it's the employee who can be in a mess, not the employer. The employer is always able to recruit in a labour market destined to overflow. Indeed, as jobs become de-skilled and technology takes over (remember BT's Directory Enquiries service), the pendulum swings in favour of the employer.

We have got to tilt the playing field in our direction, tilt the surface towards self-reliance and personal re-tooling. We need to seek new knowledge.

We are in the era of rapid product cycles. As soon as it comes on to the market there is something else to replace it. I seem to recall reading somewhere that the Sony Walkman has been redesigned 128 times in 10 years. Redesigned is perhaps the wrong word. Upgraded, remodelled, spivved up, changed. I don't know, but it does mean that technological products are as much affected by fashions as are shoes or frocks.

Cars are falling into the same category. The Volvo 400 comes in 88 different specification configurations – fashion. Owning something, whatever it is, is no longer the point; you have to own the latest model. Not good enough to have a bicycle, it has to be a mountain-bike – fashion. Computer games are fashion. The features on a mobile phone have hardly changed in five years. Sure, they've got smaller, but what they do has stayed the same. They are as much a fashion item as a damned good way of keeping in touch. And

'We are in the era of rapid product cycles. As soon as it comes on to the market there is something else to replace it. I seem to recall reading somewhere that the Sony Walkman has been redesigned 128 times in 10 years'

what can I tell parents about what we used to call plimsolls? High-tec trainers are a chimera of technology and fashion, and cost the earth.

Modern tooling means faster turn around times in bringing new products to the market and revamping old ones. New advances are driven in a curious and dangerous way, beyond our ability to control them. Research is mostly driven by curiosity and individual interest. It is an international phenomenon over which we have little say. New cures come on stream and old approaches are jettisoned. Our core products change and with them so must we: our core competencies must change as well.

> 'New advances are driven in a curious and dangerous way, beyond our ability to control them. Research is mostly driven by curiosity and individual interest. It is an international phenomenon over which we have little say'

The arena of opportunity

The future's world of work is an arena of opportunity. An arena of the new. An arena where change is the norm. An arena where it will become increasingly difficult to draw any kind of link between specific traditional skill sets, the products and services we are introducing, and the organizations we work in. We must find ways of escaping the orthodoxy of training that makes us unprepared for working in an arena of opportunity where conventional skills have become redundant. An arena of opportunity that may be impossible for some to enter and for others to exist in. Conventional training may already be redundant. Training to keep up is no good. A lifetime of continuous learning based on tomorrow's knowledge must replace reciting today what we knew yesterday.

> 'Conventional training may already be redundant'

For instance, the NHS struggles to come to grips with junior hospital doctors' hours. The veal calves of the public sector, junior hospital doctors work stupidly long hours, quite unnecessarily. Training grade doctors can work a 54 hour week. Some claim to work 70 hours. Rampant self-protectionism and political weakness prevents managers doing what they instinctively know needs to be done. Apart from reorganizing the junior doctors into a shift working system, there is an overlooked opportunity in the health arena for the nursing profession.

Ask most patients whether they would prefer to have a minor procedure carried out by an experienced ward sister three-quarters of the way through an eight-hour shift, or by a junior doctor with three weeks' experience half-way through a 70-hour week, and we know the answer. But in the NHS the customer (or patient as they still insist on calling everyone including, most irritatingly, the tax-payers who enable it all to happen), doesn't get a look in.

Arenas of opportunity exist everywhere. Dell Computers, the fast-growing hardware and software vendors, sells product back-up as an added value benefit to influence customer choice. A 'you buy the kit from us and we will help you get the best out of it' sort of deal.

I use a Toshiba laptop when travelling, but a Dell at home. I had some problems, so I called them. On-line customer service is in Ireland. So what? These days it could be on the moon. Call the number and a recorded voice (note recorded, so no costly 'hello girls' to pay), asks you a number of questions that you answer using your touch-tone telephone number pad. After several bars of musak (classicalish), a real person answers. These guys and girls speak 'several' languages and handle over 2000 calls a day from the UK alone.

Opportunity arena: get good with computers and learn another language. It is not just Dell that sells computers. We now know about the sizzling increase in PC and software sales, mostly to households whose occupants

> 'Ask most patients whether they would prefer to have a minor procedure carried out by an experienced ward sister three-quarters of the way through an eight-hour shift, or by a junior doctor with three weeks' experience half-way through a 70-hour week, and we know the answer'

can probably only get as far as opening the box without help. Helplines are here to stay. As the PC business penetrates an increasingly unsophisticated market, all kinds of teaching and helping opportunities open up a new arena.

Gateway competencies

Along the path away from the opportunity arena are gateway competencies. The labour market is bound to become congested and overflowing. As technology forces the pace of product throughput, so we will need fewer of the museums that continue to pass themselves off as workplaces, to perform our work in.

Charles Handy, the British popular business thinker reminiscent of Alfred Tack (one of the century's original management thinkers), has a vision: 'half as many people, paid twice as much, for doing three times as much' – it is a virtual reality.

In the UK's biggest remaining nationalized industry, the NHS, the past five years have seen (according to its 1994 Annual Report published by the NHS Executive): 20% of the inpatient beds go; a 50% reduction in the length of time a patient is in hospital; a 6% increase in the number of patients admitted into hospital; a 43% increase in day case admissions; and a staggering 30% increase in admissions per bed. The NHS, a political battleground, is in the British Telecom league for efficiency gains. The signs are all there, the 'Handy-Man' is right – we can do more with less.

If, in the pursuit of asset maximization, businesses merge, it is not difficult to envisage how redundancies will add up. Staff who are only just good enough will go. Staff with gateway competencies will survive.

Gateway competencies are the basis of a new deal with employers. The matriarchal deal

'...it is not difficult to envisage how redundancies will add up. Staff who are only just good enough will go. Staff with gateway competencies will survive'

between employer and employee will go. Cradle to grave welfare, training and just turning up are no good to either party. The human resource specialists and training professionals will need to rethink training, and individuals will need to train themselves in the tangential areas that conventional approaches do not embrace. Businesses want multiskilled employees. Dell, for example, needs you to be good at computers and speak another language.

A while back, something I had written in one of my magazine columns had caught the eye of the TV stations, and I spent a mad weekend doing the rounds of the TV studios. Some of the stations that wanted an interview were kind enough to send a crew to my home: two or three people – cameraman, sound recordist and a reporter.

The new cable TV news station covering the greater London area within the M25 ring came calling in the shape of just one 23-year-old. She arrived with camera, sound equipment and a list of questions, and had done the job and gone inside 20 minutes. Back at the studio she edited what she had recorded and got it on air in the lunchtime news. One person!

In New York and California you never see two-person news crews. They are all just one person. The BBC is down to two people, and as a licence-payer I'm counting!

Key to gateway competencies are computer and business skills. Computer competencies give an understanding of what technology can deliver and how to use it, instinctively, second nature.

British public services have a dreadful record on information technology (IT) procurement. Look at the foul-ups taxpayers have had to foot the bill for. These are all government IT procurement programmes that have gone 'wrong'.

'She arrived with camera, sound equipment and a list of questions, and had done the job and gone inside 20 minutes. Back at the studio she edited what she had recorded and got it on air in the lunchtime news. One person!'

- Wessex (NHS)   £64 million
- Ministry of Defence   £72 million
- Export Guarantee Scheme   £83 million
- Social Security   £44 million
- Department of Employment   £48 million

I make that £311 million – enough to run an average NHS hospital for almost four years. Ah well, back to the book… Let's try to be positive.

British public services will recover from their disastrous flirtation with IT. It will be sorted out. Messing about with benefit books when it could be done, fiddle free, with smart card technology, is just not on. Medical records could be handled in the same way. Eventually we will run out of excuses, and probably money, and someone will get on with the job of plugging government in.

The management of information through technology will not only inform businesses of how much we are doing and what it costs, but also answer questions like: does what we do work and who does it best?

This is empowerment technology; participating in a business intuitively, growing into it. Business and technology skills are gateway competencies: for a doctor in general practice, for example, this means being able to read a balance sheet with the aplomb of reading a thermometer, recognizing a business is overheating as reliably as recognizing a postoperative patient has a fever. Business diagnosis; all employees informed and able to understand where the company is going.

Gateway competencies create a chance to uncouple yourself from the traditional perceptions of colleagues, perceptions that are based on an expectation of skills that compartmentalize and truncate careers – ghettoizing the professions. Gateway competencies break into proficiencies

'The management of information through technology will not only inform businesses of how much we are doing and what it costs, but also answer questions like: does what we do work and who does it best?'

that cross professional boundaries and enable you to take a participative role in management based on sound all-round judgement.

Gateway competent managers will add skills to their repertoire. They won't wait to be trained, they will add to their own value and provide their own intellectual leadership. They will learn for themselves, become a resource centre, and be too valuable to let go: staff who can see round corners, look over the horizon, call it what you like.

Dr John Leach from Greenways Informatics reviewed my **Futureproofing** presentation at the Institute of Health Service Managers Annual Conference in Windermere in 1995, and he summed it up better than I had said it! He says that I said: 'Staff must learn to see round corners, recognizing their own skill redundancy and taking proactive steps, ahead of the game, to add value to themselves.' Thanks Doc!

Migration paths

Migration paths are the product of understanding the future. In the business environment, managing the migration path makes a lot of sense because there is always more than one path to the future. For individuals in a congested, hi-tec labour market, migration paths make more than sense – they make jobs.

Tomorrow will be full of opportunities: interactive TV; on-board navigation systems for cars as well as aeroplanes; intelligent supermarket trolleys that add up what you have purchased and make queuing at a check-out history; satellite appointment and diary management systems linked to personal communications. These are all just a taste of what we can expect. If you can imagine it – hello future. If you can't imagine it – goodbye.

Technology in health will bring us cell therapy. Cardiovascular surgery will give way to medical

> 'Staff must learn to see round corners, recognizing their own skill redundancy and taking proactive steps, ahead of the game, to add value to themselves'

interventions. Medical diagnostic services will be available in the home, and video conferencing with general practitioners (GPs) will be commonplace. The Cardiac and Data Corporation, Connecticut has developed a telediagnosis business. For example its system can spare a cardiac pacemaker-wearer a trip to hospital for a check-up. It can be done down the telephone line in seconds.

Anticipating what tomorrow's world may have for us and migrating towards it is the intelligent reaction to the uncertainty of a future that reinvents itself every day. Run to the future, don't run away from it.

The president of a Japanese investment house was asked what the most difficult part of his job was. He said it was predicting the future. He did not mean the next decade, next year, next month, next week, or even tomorrow. He said his worry was predicting what would happen in the next 10 minutes!

Futureproofing our jobs is not to define our employment as a religion, protected by a cult following of the faithful. That is dangerous talk. The world of employment is seeking to deskill, to make the job more simple.

When Mr Daimler and Mr Benz made their first motor car they *made* the motor car. I mean everything. The engine block, the chassis, they carved the pattern in the rubber tyres and did the panel beating. These boys made a car. Mr Rolls and Mr Royce did the same thing. Highly qualified people, very skilled engineers, producing, in their day, breakthrough products.

Today, motor cars that are infinitely better and more reliable are made by people who we know, from the car industry (see *page 52*) struggle to score 40% in verbal reasoning tests. Deskilling makes for better products. The evidence from the medical profession is that the more times a surgeon does an operation the better he or she gets at doing it. Stay away from general surgeons and young doctors practising late at night! Be ill during the day and live next door to a specialist in your complaint!

Deskilling jobs may be good for production, but in the long term a highly trained workforce will always win and highly trained staff have better, more transferable, job skills. Car factories that used to need 20 people to assemble a car now do it in teams of five. The teams are skilled and use robotics like you wouldn't believe. These are new skills that would be unrecognizable to Mr Rolls and Mr Benz.

Sleeping on the pavements

I don't know exactly, but it must have been more than 20 years ago that I had an experience that has stayed with me ever since. I found myself in London, near the Old Vic theatre, at about two in the morning. Outside the theatre about 50 people were sleeping on the pavement, huddled in sleeping bags and blankets.

Now, anyone visiting London today would find nothing unusual about coming across bundles sleeping in doorways. To our everlasting shame it is the norm in the 1990s. But, in the early 1970s it was an event. Curious, I made enquiries. These pavement sleepers were queuing for tickets for *Hamlet*. Richard Burton was doing his stuff and they did not want to miss it. They were sleeping on the pavement to be sure they got a ticket. They wanted to be the first in the queue when the box office opened.

It struck me, how many actors know the words to *Hamlet*? How many unemployed actors are there? Thousands of actors know the words, thousands have the professional skills to stand on the stage and do the job. But Richard Burton had that indefinable something extra that made people sleep on the pavement rather than miss it. Jimmy Connors had it, so did Torvill and Dean. My other half says George Michael has it. Who else has it?

The important question is: do you have it? Are you the sort of employee worth sleeping on the

'...how many actors know the words to *Hamlet*? How many unemployed actors are there?'

'Are you the sort of employee worth sleeping on the pavement for? Because if you're not, you could end up sleeping on the pavement yourself'

pavement for? Because if you're not, you could end up sleeping on the pavement yourself. The employment market is full of people with the right qualifications who know how to do the job. But then there is the 'third self', the indefinable bit that makes the difference.

Is it indefinable? How short of free coffee are you?

CHAPTER NINE

It's a crime, I think

Voici le soir charmant, ami du criminel.

Here is the charming evening, the criminal's friend.
Charles Baudelaire

Sometimes, some things just don't add up. Home Office crime statistics are compiled by the 43 police constabularies in England and Wales. Between July 1993 and June 1994, according to the Home Office Annual Report (published by HMSO, London 1994) 5.4 million crimes – roughly 10 crimes reported a minute, 24 hours per day, every day of the year. Seems a lot doesn't it? The fact is you are twice as likely to have your home burgled in England than in the USA. Motorists in England and Wales are more likely to have their cars stolen than motorists in the USA or most of Europe.

Expand the time frame for more than the narrow window of one year, and you find that in the five years between 1987 and 1992, property crime in England and Wales rose by an astonishing 42%.

This is all very depressing, but I fear it's not the true picture. There is probably worse to come.

The British Crime Survey (BCS), a market

> 'Between July 1993 and June 1994, the Home Office logged 5.4 million crimes.
>
> ● You are twice as likely to have your home burgled in England than in the USA
>
> ● Motorists in England and Wales are more likely to have their car stolen than motorists in the USA or most of Europe'

research approach based on 14 000 interviews, logged 18 million acts of crime between 1993 and 1994 – a big difference from the Home Office Statistics for the same period. What is the explanation?

I think the BCS results are probably nearer the truth. BCS found that only 41% of the victims of crime had bothered to report it to the police. BCS found that the reasons for not reporting crime included: victims not wishing to see their insurance premiums increase; loss of no claims bonus; and the acceptance of higher levels of 'excess', the amount of a loss that must be met by the insured.

'The British Crime Survey (BCS), a market research approach based on 14 000 interviews, logged 18 million acts of crime'

Very significantly, another reason was a lack of confidence that 'it was worth bothering to report' crimes, as 'no one gets caught'. Some police forces (strange how we think of the police as a 'force' and not a 'service'), have changed the way in which they record crime.

For example, in some areas, if a burglar attempts to break into your property and fails the crime is recorded as 'wilful damage', which is a civil matter, not a crime! That keeps the numbers down.

The extent to which crime affects the economy is hard to estimate, but let me tell you about a simple offence of breaking and entering.

A friend of mine had been out at work all day and came home to find the back gate had been forced, a panel of glass on the back door had been broken, the lock busted and the wooden doorframe split.

There was mud all over the carpets, and the video had been yanked out of the wall, damaging the socket and the leads into and out of the TV. For good measure, the cabinet that housed the video had been scratched.

The bills my friend had to fork out for are shown in Table 5.

Table 5 The cost of a simple break-in

Item	Replacement cost (£)	
Repair and replace back gate, lock and fence post	45	
Back door glass	8	(temporary repair)
Fitting back door glass	15	(temporary repair)
New back door lock	45	
Repairs to door frame and redecoration	105	
Clean carpet	80	
French polish cabinet	95	
Repairs and replacements to aerial and power leads to TV/video	65	
Replace video	400	
Total	858	

Now, this tidy little sum does not take account of the endless 'phone calls, time off work and the cost of a burglar alarm!

Let's look at the other side of the balance sheet. What was the gain to the little so-and-so who caused my friend so much grief? I am told, by those who know about these things, that a hot (stolen) video can be 'fenced' (sold to a third party) for about £40.

In the circumstances, you can see why victims don't bother telling anyone. It is most unlikely anyone will be caught. Letting on to your insurers puts up your premiums and loses you your no claims bonus. The burglar alarm? Forget it. Because of the number of false alarms the police have to deal with they have announced they are scaling down their response to them.

The best idea I have for my friend is not a 100% foolproof anticrime suggestion, but it might just work all the same. Take a £50 note, put it in an envelope and tape it to the back door with a note:

> *Dear Mr Burglar*
>
> *Save us all a lot of grief, take the fifty quid and leave my house alone.*
>
> *Yours faithfully*
> *Grateful Home Owner*

I am sure my friends in the police will not be too pleased about the idea. However, they do have some explaining to do. My friend is very unlikely to see her video again, and if she does it is more likely to be the result of geography than detective work. Table 6 shows why.

Wales seems to be a safer place to live than Humberside, which looks like an expensive, risky proposition – there is a 25.2 percentage point difference between detected crime in Dyfed and Humberside. What is it like in your area? Where I live, more than three-quarters of offenders appear to get away with it. Is it any wonder the insurance companies are putting up their rates?

Police forces in some areas solve twice as many crimes as others. The Audit Commission noted that the forces likely to catch the most criminals were the ones that targeted their efforts, focusing on known criminals, and had civilians to handle the paperwork.

> 'Police forces in some areas solve twice as many crimes as others ... the forces likely to catch the most criminals were the ones that targeted their efforts, focusing on known criminals, and had civilians to handle the paperwork'

Table 6 Crime detection rate and cost*

Constabulary	Crimes detected by primary means (%)	Cost per head of population (£)
Dyfed-Powys	40.5	88.26
Gwent	35.1	91.86
Lincolnshire	33.7	90.24
Wiltshire	33.6	91.77
North Wales	28.3	90.40
Cumbria	27.5	104.61
Suffolk	27.4	84.26
Dorset	27	86.39
Durham	25.4	86.42
Lancashire	25.3	97.74
Merseyside	25.1	140.06
Northamptonshire	25	90.15
North Yorkshire	24.9	85.30
Cleveland	24.4	111.44
Norfolk	24.3	82.20
Cheshire	23.9	76.43
Essex	23.9	90.66
Hampshire and Isle of Wight	22.7	83.30
Devon and Cornwall	22.4	90.48
Staffordshire	22.2	89.77
West Mercia	22.2	81.25
Kent	21.9	92.86
Surrey	21.8	97.12
Nottinghamshire	21.5	93.46
Cambridgeshire	20.7	81.72
Sussex	20.6	83.88
Hertfordshire	20	85.66
Northumbria	19.1	110.75
South Wales	18.9	101.16
Derbyshire	18.7	82.60
Leicestershire	18.5	84.10
Warwickshire	18.2	93.37
Thames Valley	18	89.33
Metropolitan Police	17.7	228.45
Gloucestershire	17.1	92.38
Bedfordshire	17	94
Greater Manchester	17	117.73
South Yorkshire	16.8	99.19
West Midlands	16.8	108.62
West Yorkshire	16.4	108.39
Avon and Somerset	15.5	92.17
Humberside	15.3	100.98

*Source: Audit Commission's Survey of Police Forces in England and Wales 1995.

In the language of business, the successful forces were the ones who had *re-engineered* their processes, changed and adapted what they do in the light of changing circumstances. **Futureproofed**. The police call the process civilianization, employing civilians to carry out work previously performed by the police officers themselves. Everyone that I know in the police force manages to pronounce the word 'civilianization' as though they were saying the 'end of civilization'. It is not popular, and there has been a lot of opposition to it within the police. However, the success of re-engineering speaks for itself. (For the civilian, the police force has become an opportunity arena for gateway competencies.)

As we look into the future, there is nothing that predicts or gives us reason to believe that, in the long run, crime rates will fall. The greater use of electronic devices such as burglar and car alarms will create fast track product development but will shift the emphasis of crime from one sector to another. In 1995, for example, violent offences against people increased, but crime against property fell. And, you can't fix a burglar alarm to people.

The police services (better word!) up and down the country will be looking for more resources and the pressure will be to get more for less. Some police officers are already asking radical questions. If you are daft enough to leave an unattended briefcase in full view of the back seat of your car, should the police bother to look for the thief who will steal it? If a house is broken into and there were inadequate locks or no burglar alarm, should the police have to investigate the crime? Almost all property can be protected and almost all property crime can be avoided – should we continue to expect the police service to look after the things that we are careless about? These are tough questions and they get asked because resources are not elastic. The real question is how do we make every police service as good as the best and get everyone's results in line?

This is not healthy

The same geographic variables are at play in the NHS as in the police: where you live is the most important factor in whether you can obtain quick and satisfactory treatment. In the language of the manager, outcomes are variable.

Think about walking into a branch of McDonalds and asking for a Big Mac. Whether you live in Brighton or Birmingham, Manchester or Margate, Sheffield or Singapore, Yorkshire or New York, you would expect to eat a sesame seed bun, an all-beef patty, relish and all the other goodies, and you will be sure to get it.

Think about flying British Airways to Washington DC. Wherever you board the flight – Gatwick, Heathrow, Manchester – you still arrive in the right place.

Consistency of outcomes – a great way to run a business.

It's not too much to ask is it?

The problems in the NHS are well illustrated by Table 7, which gives figures for the health services in Scotland.

When the figures were published by the Scottish Office, the health

Table 7 Patient survival rates of heart attack in Scotland*

	Number of patients admitted	Died within 30 days	Mortality rate (%)
Top five hospitals			
Western General	1032	165	15.47
Borders General	786	132	16.31
Dundee Teaching	2371	427	17.74
West Glasgow University	2133	370	17.83
Aberdeen Royal	2547	438	18.10
Five lowest rate			
Fife Healthcare	886	292	29.56
Grampian Healthcare	471	190	26.54
Royal Alexandra	1398	338	25.68
Argyle and Bute	496	134	25.01
Law Hospital	1404	330	24.81

*Source: Clinical Outcome Indicators Scotland, December 1994.

establishment went potty. Mr Jim Johnson, chairman of the British Medical Association (BMA) consultants' group, dismissed the tables as 'irresponsible' because patients would be worried if they were sent to a hospital with a low rating. Too right Mr Johnson! I don't want to go to one with a poor rating, thank you! Health bosses argued that the indicators did not take account of the fact that some patients might have other things wrong with them that could exacerbate their illnesses and make a recovery less viable. OK, I won't argue with that. But can someone explain why there is a 14% difference between one hospital and another within the same region?

The *Guardian* newspaper wasn't too impressed either. An editorial on 21 June 1994 said:

> After school league tables, stand by for the Government's 'good hospitals guide': a hotel-style ratings system designed to provide the public with a quick-glance to the performance of their local hospitals. Predictably, MPs from both main opposition parties (as well as the BMA) are lining up to make fools of themselves.

> All the predictable criticisms were being trotted out yesterday: the impossibility of the task, its unfairness – and the distortions it would create. The opposition of the BMA is understandable. They have a professional conspiracy to defend. But opposition MPs should stop denying patients – and the public – important information which they have a democratic right to know.

> No one was making the real criticism: meekness of the Government's so-called radical proposal, and its refusal to tackle the real issues – mortality and morbidity tables. All opponents should be asked one question. *If you were having to parachute from a plane tomorrow and you knew that one parachute packer never made a mistake but the other had a 20% error rate, would you want to know who had packed your chute?*

Too right! And the outcomes saga in the NHS gets worse.

William Windham became famous as the Secretary of War against revolutionary France. He lived in Norfolk. In 1810 he went to help a neighbour whose library was on fire. Big panic (no CD-ROM back-up in those days). Poor old Bill fell off the ladder and broke his hip. He was operated on and died a few days later. End of a great man.

Here we are 185 years later, and people in East Anglia are still dying after their hips have been operated on. The *British Medical Journal* reported a survey of the differences in outcomes of 500 broken hips in various hospitals in the area.

The patients were admitted to eight different hospitals. All the hospitals were used to dealing with this type of injury and the areas patients came from had no huge differences in socioeconomic or deprivation factors. The patients' age, sex and occupations were all very similar.

And that's where the similarities ended. The death rate in the first 90 days after surgery varied from 5–24%.

All sorts of oddities emerged from the study: 245 of the operations were postponed for 24 hours, and in 192 of these cases there were no grounds for delay.

After an operation all kinds of nasty things can happen: wound infections, pulmonary embolism, deep vein thrombosis and heart attacks. In this study, women had a three times better survival rate than men. The biggest factors seemed to be that anticoagulants and antibiotics were not used as a matter of routine in some hospitals. Early mobilization and early surgery were also important for a good outcome.

In layman's terms: some hospitals didn't get on with the job fast enough or do the job thoroughly enough. If granny dies after a hip replacement and she wasn't operated on early enough, prescribed antibiotic cover or anticoagulatnts, and was not got mobile fast enough, who (apart from granny, of course) suffers the consequences? The relatives, not the doctor.

Most doctors live a largely sanction-free existence because they have turned what they do into an impenetrable mystery so that no one can

'The death rate in the first 90 days after surgery varied from 5–24%. All sorts of oddities emerged from the study: 245 of the operations were postponed for 24 hours, and in 192 of these cases there were no grounds for delay'

'In layman's terms: some hospitals didn't get on with the job fast enough or do the job thoroughly enough'

challenge them. The government has introduced a Bill into the House of Commons that, if enacted, will compel errant doctors to face assessment and possible retraining. The Medical (Professional Performance) Bill has all-party support. Think about it, a law to force people to do the job they're paid to do – a crazy world. And we pay for it all!

If the East Anglia survey is typical of the UK as a whole, half of the 55 000 patients admitted to hospital each year with a broken hip will not receive anticoagulants and quite a few of them will not be operated on straight away.

We are talking about people's lives here – not a McDonalds. Let's get a plane away from all this insanity!

Flight of fancy

In the USA, 5–10% of all flight delays are due to mechanical problems. The Transportation Department intended to publish league tables about the delays. Consumer groups got excited and everyone was ready. It didn't happen. Why? Good question. The authorities received three complaints about what was proposed and decided against doing it.

> 'In the USA, 5–10% of all flight delays are due to mechanical problems. The Transportation Department intended to publish league tables about the delays. Consumer groups got excited and everyone was ready. It didn't happen. Why?'

Three complaints! They were from Northwest Airlines, Southwest Airlines and America Airways. Enough said? They said that by publishing 'late flight' information, employees would be likely to rush through repairs for the sake of a good on-time record and safety could be compromised. Whatever happened to process control?

We've looked at three organizations. The police and the NHS in the UK, and the USA's internal air transport. None of them has consistent outcomes, all of them resist being measured and no one wants to tell us anything. How do you fancy being an airline passenger, taken ill on the way home and arrive to find your house has been broken into?

Wellington said 'publish and be damned'; he was talking about something else but he could just as well have been talking about how not to run an organization. Unless we measure what we do, calibrate it, benchmark it, how will we know if we are any good? More importantly, how will our customers know? Organizations of the future won't exist on fog or fudge. If you are any good tell people – if you're not, get out of the game.

CHAPTER TEN **Goose bump good**

Tous les jours, à tous points de vue, je vais de mieux en mieux

Every day, in every way, I am getting better and better
Émile Coué

What business are you in? Its not a bad question. Ask most people what business they are in and they will get the answer wrong; they have no idea. They may know where they work, they may know what they do when they get there, but they will have no idea what business they are in.

Alan Jones, chief executive officer of the logistics company TNT, knows exactly what business he is in. Picking up packages and delivering them to the right place is not a bad description of the TNT business. Having a fleet of huge lorries that don't breakdown is not a bad start. Carting stuff around at competitive prices is attractive. It's all wrong. Alan Jones will tell you he is in the 'absolutely, positively, get it there overnight, in one piece or die' business.

> 'Alan Jones will tell you he is in the "absolutely, positively, get it there overnight, in one piece or die" business'

What business is a restaurant in? As sure as eggs is eggs it is not in the food business. It might be in the fast food business, like Burger King or McDonalds; perhaps the romantic evening business, like the Caprice, in London's Mayfair; or the Greek business, like the little place you found on holiday; the Chinese business, like Hyns in South Ascot – visit there and I will probably be at my usual table by the window near the big white grand piano that they play jazz on three nights a week.

Whatever restaurants do, wherever they are, they are not in the food business. We don't visit just for food. We visit for the atmosphere, the speed of service, the dancing, the music, the price, oh, and then the food. The meat of the business is not what it does. It is not the steak we are interested in, it's the sizzle.

What business is the NHS in? Is it in the 'when granny falls over in the high street and breaks the neck of her femur, let's give her a prosthetic hip' business? No, I think not. The NHS should be in the 'can we get granny back on her feet in time to get down to the Day Centre, fit and ready for her birthday party knees-up?' business. The NHS is not in the maternity business – it is in the generation game. The NHS is in the 'how fast can we safely get you back to work to earn a living' business.

Out of town shopping complexes are in the 'shopping can be fun' and 'leisure' businesses; the software industry is in the load it up and use it to get the job done' business. What business are you in? The question matters. And it probably matters more than any other question we might ask ourselves about the future of the organizations we run, work with and try to hang on to.

The answer to the question is the strategic mission of the business and its quality statement.

Count Helmuth von Moltke's revolutionary approach to strategy won the Austro-Prussian War in 1866, and for good measure he did it again five years later, in the Franco-Prussian War in 1871. To an army used to being told what to do down to the nth degree he said: 'strategy is applied common sense and cannot be taught'. He never gave direct orders, he gave directives and left autonomous officers to get on with the job of winning the war. They did not need to be told the war could not be won without winning the battles on the way.

All my friends who have swatted up on strategy in

> 'What business are you in? The question matters. And it probably matters more than any other question we might ask ourselves about the future of the organizations we run, work with and try to hang on to'

business in their later years and given up weekend parties and holidays to achieve their Masters Degree in Business Administration (MBA), will cross me off their Christmas card list. But, it has to be said, I agree with Helmuth. Strategy cannot be taught, and even if it could be, it would be average strategy because education is about achieving the highest possible average pass.

Strategy is intuitive; it's a feeling; it's about knowing that granny wants to get home as fast as she can, to get on with her life, because that's what we would want if we were granny.

Defining what business we are in is the first and last step we need to take to encapsulate our mission, our values and the quality of our goods and services. It is the only strategic statement we need to make and it must be congenital – bred into the business and part of the genes of everyone who works there.

> **'I agree with Helmuth. Strategy cannot be taught, and even if it could be, it would be average strategy because education is about achieving the highest possible average pass'**

If you can develop an organization dedicated to a constant sense of change, and you will need to just to survive, the quality of what you do is the only ticket you can buy to get into the future arena and play the game by the new rules of the future. Quality must be like the stripe in the toothpaste and run all the way through strategy; strategy must run through quality like the weft of fine plaid.

Quality. I hate using the word. I hate talking about it. After all, quality is only about getting people to do what they come to work to do, right first time, every time. When people talk quality I wonder what they are hiding.

How many times have I seen quality worn like a bandage, a war wound carried home from the front line of contact with the customer? Quality, stuck like a go-faster stripe on the side of an ageing saloon. Quality, sprayed around like an air freshener in the men's changing room. I am bored with quality, fed up to the back teeth with it, and I make it a rule never to discuss it.

OK, you talked me into it. I will break my rule and discuss quality for one last time.

Look, quality doesn't matter any more. Quality has had it. If you still have to talk about quality, get out of the business because the caravan has moved on and only the dogs are left barking. If you have got a quality problem, close down because as sure as hell you won't catch up.

The NHS still talks about quality, God help it. It still has to do 9% of all hip operations twice; some doctors say half of all hysterectomies aren't worth doing (they just don't know which half); and the outcome variations on breast cancer are about as varied as the performance of the 43 police forces in England and Wales (see page 70). The NHS and the police forces are the dying embers of the final days of the nationalized industry. Give them 10 years and they will have gone the same way as the coal industry or British Airways – I can't quite decide which! (*See next book, Ed.*)

> 'Quality, stuck like a go-faster stripe on the side of an ageing saloon. Quality, sprayed around like an air freshener in the men's changing room. I am bored with quality, fed up to the back teeth with it, and I make it a rule never to discuss it'

Everybody else has got it. They have cottoned on. No quality, no business. The Japanese can throw together the 8000 parts it needs to make a car, or a hi-fi, or a computer, or an oven, or a wristwatch, or a satellite navigation system or whatever, with *zero* quality defects.

Quality is taken for granted. German cars don't break down. Spanish onions don't have bugs in them and French apples don't have maggots. People, passengers, shoppers, consumers – they don't want to know about quality. They take it for granted.

When the high-tec high aspiration Eurostar trains break down, passengers get off, get their money back, and go by boat next time. Consumers are cruel. If Marks and Spencer sells something that doesn't fit or fouls up, it will change it or refund your money, no question, and hope you will go back. Mostly we do. Customers can be forgiving, too, if you treat them right.

No one can afford to take a gamble on quality. Even the emerging industrial nations realize quality is not a bolt-on, it is a bolt-up or belt off. Look out for the Pacific rim nations as they break into Western markets. The last thing they bother with is quality – they have done all that already, it was the first thing they did. By the time they get to you quality is routine.

Quality no longer sells products. Without quality, products just don't sell – it's as simple as that. Make poor quality stuff, lose customers, get sued and go to gaol. Poor quality raises hackles and good quality no longer raises goose bumps. No, we need something else.

What do we do to be different? In a world where quality ceases to be a differential, at a time when the best is routine, what do we do? What is next, beyond quality? Price? No, everyone has to keep prices to a minimum. Consumers expect bargains and given a choice, they just go somewhere else. Where will the goose bumps come from?

> 'Quality no longer sells products. Without quality, products just don't sell – it's as simple as that. Make poor quality stuff, lose customers, get sued and go to gaol. Poor quality raises hackles and good quality no longer raises goose bumps. No, we need something else'

Grease is the word!

Beyond quality is Grease! It is hard to imagine but it's true. If you are a contemporary of mine you will know exactly what I mean. *Grease!* the musical. 'Grease!' Remember the words? 'Grease is the word; it's got groove; it's got meaning. Grease is the time, it's the place, it's the motion. Grease is the way we are feeling today.' Grease is exciting. It's electrifying!

Grease is what is beyond boring, every one the same, never goes wrong, made five million of them working within a millisecond of each other, quality. Something exciting. Swatch Watches are quality, they tell the time, don't go wrong (quality) and they are fun, fashion, status and Grease! Tie Rack ties are fine quality silk and they are Grease! Body Shops are quality and Grease! The Planet Hollywood Restaurant chain is Grease!

Futureproofed organizations are Grease! Organizations need to be exciting, not just for the people who work in them but for the users and customers, too. Getting your parcel from Ipswich to Inverness *'absolutely, positively, get it there overnight, in one piece or die'* is exciting. It is exciting for Alan Jones who leads the company, for the staff who do it and the customers who pay for it. More than quality it is the corporate challenge, the excitement. Working in McDonalds as part of the front of house crew (and I have done it) is exhausting, but it is exciting.

Getting granny to the Day Centre party is the only quality test worth applying to the NHS. The granny test – that's exciting. Exciting for the doctors and nurses who achieve it and the relatives who will see it happen. Getting granny's hip right first time is exciting.

Helmuth von Moltke must have been an exciting guy to work for and he and his troops were winners. And what else is there but winning?

'Swatch Watches are quality, they tell the time, don't go wrong (quality) and they are fun (Grease!). Tie Rack ties are fine quality silk and they are Grease! Body Shops are quality and Grease! The Planet Hollywood Restaurant chain is Grease!'

Exciting is mission, it is value, it is strategy and it is motivation for everyone in and around the organization – it is Grease! And it is goose-bump good.

CHAPTER ELEVEN

Faith, dope and charity

Hope is a good breakfast, but it is a bad supper
Francis Bacon

The British Crime Survey (BCS) (see page 67) that showed up such a difference between Home Office statistics and people's experiences of crime has another surprise for us. The 18 million acts of crime it logged in the 1993/94 period did not include drugs offences.

Rough calculations suggest that we would need to spend upwards of £350 million per year on law enforcement if we are to have a significant impact on the drugs problem. A further £165 million is needed by the NHS to provide its complex network of GPs, clinics, acute services, detoxification programmes, counselling and needle exchange services. That adds up to £515 million, or just over £15 per head of the working population. You may say that this is a great deal of money, and you would be right. But it is a tiny amount taken against what some say is the value of the drugs industry as a whole.

Journalists write about the 'drugs industry' (for that is what it has become – a business) and, borrowing phrases from the business pages, some even try to value its turnover; they say it's 'worth' over £3 billion. Far fetched? Who knows. Estimates put drug related property crime to be 'worth' £5 billion. Worth, value, turnover. Back streets have become Wall Street; inner-city crime translates into the language of the City of London. Assets are human lives and turnover too bleak to define.

> 'In 1994, the UK spent £350 million on drugs enforcement. Treatment for people addicted to drugs costs about £165 million per year. Drugs-related property crime is estimated to be worth £5 billion'

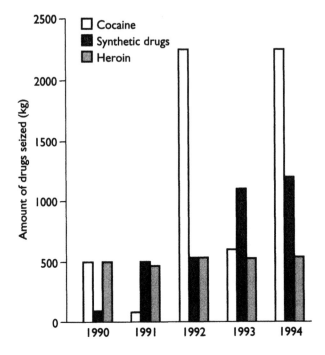

Figure 6 UK drugs seizures. (Source: Her Majesty's Customs and Excise, 1994.)

As drugs and drugs related crimes take more and more of a toll, costing the taxpayer dear in terms of policing and health services, the question pushing its way to the top of the agenda is: should some drugs be decriminalized or even legalized?

The interesting point to make about the statistics (Figure 6) is the inconsistencies there are in the seizure figures and the lingering, unanswered question: if this is what they catch, how much slips through unnoticed?

See there's that word again, 'inconsistencies'.

In 1994, the amount of cocaine seized by customs officials rose by 224%, and a record amount of other drugs was seized as well. All told, it amounted to about 51 tonnes of drugs.

Mike King, of the National Union of Civil and
Public Services Association, is quoted as saying: 'All
the evidence leads drug experts to conclude that
despite the success of drugs seizures, drugs are still
flooding into the UK in unprecedented quantities.'

> 'All the
> evidence leads
> drug experts
> to conclude
> that despite
> the success of
> drugs seizures,
> drugs are still
> flooding into
> the UK in
> unprecedented
> quantities'

Would you like to see my etchings?

I was at a charity lunch. It was coming to an end,
thank goodness: too much booze and too much
food. A couple of hundred of the great and the
good raising money for a drugs rehabilitation
something or other. I had been too self-indulgent
by half. I had swallowed all my holiday promises
to cut down and cut out. My mind wandered and I was fed up, literally.

The woman sitting next to me leaned forward, asked me if I would like to
see her etchings! I agreed and we made for her apartment.

She was as good as her word. The etchings were
some of the finest I have seen. Engravings by
Cruikshank, first published in the *Gentleman's
Pocket Magazine* in the late 1800s. She was a
serious collector: pictures of Dickens' London;
the *Hackney Coachman*, the *Chimney Sweeper*,
Turncock and the Beadle, and a collection of
meticulous etchings of characters from London's
gin palaces. Lives ruined by mother's ruin;
tortured folk who drank their wages and stole
for the rest; images of a time when a glass of gin
cost half a week's wages and of the men and
women who lived squalid lives because of it.

> 'After a robust
> exchange of my
> Anglo-Saxon
> and his
> Glaswegian, I
> soon realized
> that questions
> such as "What
> the hell are you
> doing here?"
> were not the
> most tactful
> in the
> circumstances'

As I left her apartment building and was about
to step into the bright lights of a rain soaked
West End, I tripped over a bundle in the
entrance way and went sprawling. The bundle

moved, and from beneath a pile of stinking blankets a head popped out. This, I was later to discover, was Ian. After a robust exchange of my Anglo-Saxon and his Glaswegian, I soon realized that questions such as 'What the hell are you doing here?' were not the most tactful in the circumstances.

I was curious. Somehow I found myself in the nearby McDonalds, stumping up for two coffees and a burger. Ian told me he had come to London from Glasgow in search of work. He had discovered that there was, is and will ever be, only one Dick Whittington, and life is not a pantomime.

Unemployment, family rows and a fierce pride had prevented him from going home and was the start of a spiral of decline.

A chance meeting in a pub had brought him into contact with some new friends. They had cheered him up, bought him a few drinks and invited him to a party. His introduction to 'smack' (heroin to you and me) was at a party. At first it was a gift to help get him in the party mood; then he was asked to 'contribute a few quid because the stuff doesn't grow on trees'. Then the price went up, and within a month it was spiralling in direct proportion to his craving.

The rest is a bleak personal history. Ian spends the mornings shoplifting and stealing from cars, the afternoons peddling the stolen goods to the 'fences', the 'thieving buggers who pay peanuts for good gear', and the evenings in the King's Cross area of London with the pimps, prostitutes and pushers, in search of a fix to see him through the night.

Even if he had the cash, Ian could not get a hostel place. They turn away junkies because the junkies can turn nasty. 'What about a cure?' I asked. Another tactless gaffe on my part. Ian had tried

'As society cracks up, we can only help pick up the pieces. In 1994, seizures of "crack cocaine" alone went up by 370%, a silent killer that weighs tonnes and kills in grams. In the whole of the UK there are only 108 doctors who have Home Office permission to prescribe cocaine'

getting by on methadone, but like most junkies he had ended up selling it to raise the cash to buy some real drugs.

Dr John Marks is a consultant psychiatrist at a drugs dependency clinic in Cheshire. His radical approach to drug dependency is not unlike that taken by one of his famous predecessors, a certain Dr Petro, who in the 1970s could be found, by those in the know, in miserable consulting rooms in the back streets of Waterloo in London. He dispensed drugs on prescription to drug addicts. The medical establishment was not ready for Dr Petro. As I recall, he got struck off for his trouble.

How Dr Marks will fair I don't know. He argues that his approach will cut down the risk of HIV infection and undermine the market value of illegal drugs. He is trying to deal with the moral conundrum that anyone could trip over in the doorway of some posh flats in London.

Dr Marks is prescribing heroin and cocaine to dozens of patients, including some on 'crack', the smokeable form of cocaine that is absorbed into the bloodstream much more quickly and is altogether a much more vicious drug.

The benefits, he claims, are obvious. Undermine the value of the drugs market, save the rest of us from outbreaks of petty (and sometimes not so petty) crime, reduce the spread of HIV and other infections, and enable users to have half a chance of getting a job and maintaining relationships, maybe even getting off the stuff. The disadvantages are running the risk of psychotic behaviour among addicts.

As society cracks up, we can only help pick up the pieces. In 1994, seizures of 'crack cocaine' alone went up by 370%, a silent killer that weighs tonnes and kills in grams. In the whole of the UK there are only 108 doctors who have Home Office permission to prescribe cocaine. One of them has been prevented from prescribing and a private doctor in London has been charged with 18 counts of prescribing drugs 'irresponsibly'. Dr Petro, déjà vu. The rest of the profession appears to struggle by prescribing methadone.

'In some areas of the UK, drugs-related crime accounts for half the offences committed'

In some areas of the UK, drugs-related crime accounts for half the offences committed. It is difficult not to conclude that drugs-related crime will soon be out of control.

For every drugs bust we see reported, tonnes of drugs slip into circulation behind our backs. We all suffer the consequences. By the time they are 15 years old, half the children in the UK will have experimented with some form of illegal substance.

> 'By the time they are 15 years old, half the children in the UK will have experimented with some form of illegal substance'

Today, newspapers and TV describe the reality that Cruikshank once engraved. Legalization, sensible controls and licensing wiped out the squalor of the gin palaces. I wonder how many more charity lunches there will be and how many more Ians, before we lose faith in the drugs enforcement agencies and start a real debate about licensing the sale of drugs.

That makes the future a really dangerous place.

The UK is growing older

A friend of mine has a delightful pub tucked away in the South Downs. Oak beams, wooden floors and horse brasses, you know the kind of thing. He is a jolly fellow with a great sense of humour. He and his wife are the ideal couple to run a pub.

He tells the story of one evening when three elderly people came into the bar, a woman and two men. One of the men approached the bar and ordered two gin and tonics and a pint of free beer. 'Free beer!', said my landlord friend. 'You must be joking.' 'Oh,' said the sprightly grey haired man at the bar, 'you must give me a free pint. Look at your sign.'

He pointed to a sign behind the bar that reads:

FREE BEER

For everyone over 65 years old accompanied by both parents

The grey haired man continued: 'I am 65 years old and I would like you to meet my parents, Doris and Bill, who are aged 83 years and 85 years respectively!'

My landlord friend stumped up the free pint and has since taken the notice down! Risky sign – we are getting older.

The UK's so-called ageing population is a well known concern, not just to my landlord friend. The NHS is struggling with government policies that seek to disengage long-term care from the health service and push it towards the social services (where the costs can be means-tested) and greater individual self-reliance. The policy, undoubtedly Treasury driven, is not without a rationale. Admissions of elderly people to hospital are increasing at the rate of about 4% per annum. To keep pace with demographic changes, a 0.7% increase in spending on health for the over 65s is needed. If service trends are taken into account, the figure rises to 1.2%.

To bring the increase in spending into sharp focus, in 1994, the increase, in real money terms, on expenditure for the NHS was 1.5%. If increases remain at the same level, demand will inevitably outstrip resources. Figures which highlight this are shown in Figure 7.

Staying in hospital costs money, and the old are living longer. Before the First World War life expectancy was under 55 years; today the figure has rocketed to 72 years for men and 78 years for women.

As people live longer, they often get sicker. Three out of four of those aged 80 or over suffer from some form of mental or physical disability.

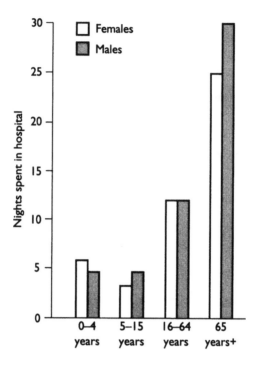

Figure 7 Number of nights spent in hospital in 1993. (Source: Office of Population Censuses and Surveys.)

In 1993, there were something like 800 000 patients suffering from Alzheimer's disease and a further 100 000 suffering from Parkinson's disease in the UK.

We are simply, not getting any younger (Figure 8).

In 1992 we spent 1.5% of our gross domestic product (GDP) on continuing care for the elderly. By 2000, projections put it at 3.5%.

Paying for continuing care is a headache for both the state and individuals. In 1994, 40 000 elderly couples were forced to sell their houses in order to pay the bills for continuing care.

Old does not always mean poor, but the indications are that it generally does (Figure 9).

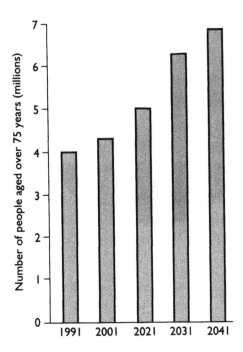

Figure 8 Projection of how the population of the UK will age to 2041. (Source: Office of Population Censuses and Surveys.)

Encouraging people to make greater personal provision for their old age is likely to become a feature of political policy-making and to result in a range of new products from the insurance, savings and pension industries.

The 'baby-boom' generation reaches retirement in 20 years' time and will place intolerable strains on health and social service agencies. Today's savings programmes won't help as much as they could. Money invested in Tessas and Personal Equity Plans does not attract tax relief, only the interest earned is tax-free. New plans aimed at encouraging individuals to make greater provision for their old age are likely to attract tax relief on entry and exit.

The USA, facing the same sorts of problems, has already made changes to its savings tax structure. Americans can enjoy tax benefits if they invest in

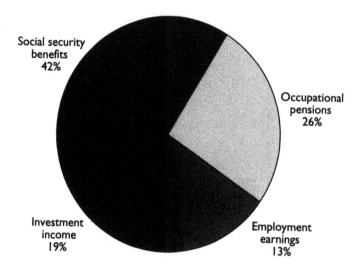

Figure 9 Pensioners' sources of income. (Source: Social Trends, 1995.)

individual savings schemes tailored especially for retirement. The schemes also allow an early hypothecated withdrawal for the purchase of the first home and for university education and health care.

A similar sort of scheme operates in Singapore. Germany is now requiring individuals to make special provision to pay the bills for the care of the elderly.

Cruising

So, the world is getting greyer and the outlook is a bit grey too. Making provision for our old age is a sensible thing to do. The pictures on TV of ideal couples walking ideal dogs into the sunset, or standing on the deck of a cruise ship, are just about everyone's idea of happy retirement. But can it be done?

In his book *The State We're In* (Jonathan Cape, London, 1995), Will Hutton makes the point that the size of your pension depends on the product of two factors: how much you have stashed away, and how well it has been invested.

The process is simple enough. You give your cash to the pensions company, which invests it for you, generally in the 200 or so blue chip companies in the UK stock market, with a few overseas investments and maybe some gold or diamonds for good measure.

When you are ready to retire, the investments are cashed in and you buy an annuity which gives you an income stream for the rest of your days and pays for the cruise, the daughter's wedding, and keeps the dog in Fido meat.

> 'The pictures on TV of ideal couples walking ideal dogs into the sunset, or standing on the deck of a cruise ship, are just about everyone's idea of happy retirement. But can it be done?'

The yield on the annuity is the important point. They have been around 9% for some time, so, for the purposes of the example, let's stay with that. If you want a pension of, say, £13 000 a year (an extrapolation from the 1995 Social Trends Survey puts average gross weekly earnings at about £326 per week, or just on £17 000 per year), you will have to accumulate a pension annuity fund of about £150 000.

Let's take a look into the crystal ball. We know that earnings are growing at about 3% a year, and the stock market puts on about 8–8.5% growth each year. So, without inflation (because that makes the sum too difficult for me!), I reckon you will have to save just over £3000 a year, or £60 a week.

And there is one more thing you need to take into account. By the time the baby-boomers have got to retirement age there will be about 12 million of them, and they will all be looking to do the same thing.

I'm not sure how big the fund would have to be to pay all those pension-boomers what they want, but it would have to be about £2 billion. I guess we would have to more than double the UK's performance and national output to achieve that kind of growth. Anyway, saving £60 a week, week in week out, is probably impossible on a national average income of

£17 000, which after tax and national insurance slides down to £14 000.

OK, so **Futureproof** that lot! Understanding how the pensions industry works is a good start. If the day you sell your pension assets the stock market is having a funny five minutes, you lose. Choose a pension fund manager that sells your shares over a period, to avoid a big bang or a big bust. Yields on annuities vary, shop around; ask the pension fund administrators how they see the annuity market; ask the questions well before your fund matures; become an expert in pensions.

> 'If the day you sell your pension assets the stock market is having a funny five minutes, you lose'

For the longer term, it seems clear to me that the numbers simply do not add up. Welfare is wealth – that's the message.

Family life

As the UK grows older, so there are social and other age changes. The UK's families are changing and changing fast. The concept of family and marriage has taken on a whole new look.

As usual, while the politicians are talking about one thing, everyone else is doing the opposite! Families seem to me to be disappearing fast.

An increasing percentage of children are being born into households where either the parents are not married, or one parent is missing (Figure 10). There is no moral or philosophical point to be made here – just a good old practical one. If single parents are busy looking after the kids, how do they work and where does the money come from?

Looking after a couple of kids alone does not make work easy for the majority who are undereducated and have few job prospects. Day to day survival puts further education, retraining and child care out of reach. The Treasury takes the strain.

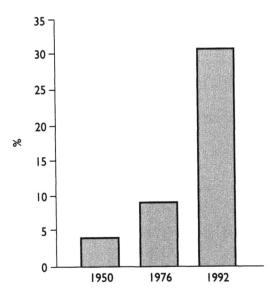

Figure 10 How the percentage of children born outside marriage in the UK has changed. (Source: *CSJ*, 1994.)

Of the 31% of children born outside marriage, 55% have two parents in the household. The catch is that 50% of cohabitations last only two years, and 16% for only five years. The number of lone parents is increasing, and the number of lone parent households has almost tripled in the past 30 years (Figure 11).

The full breakdown of how families in the UK are made up is shown in Figure 12.

Until the mid-1980s, the gradual increase in the proportion of lone mothers was mainly caused by an increase in the number of divorced mothers. During the mid-1980s the increase was more rapid so that now one in five mothers with dependent children is a lone mother. The proportion of lone fathers has changed little at under 2% of all families. For some reason the divorce lawyers had a field day in 1981!

Table 8 throws up some weird anomalies, mainly due to marriage rates.

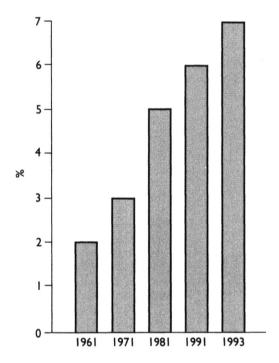

Figure 11 Percentage of UK households of lone parents with dependent children. Total UK households = 22.9 million. (Source: Office of Population Censuses and Surveys, Department of the Environment, Scottish Office Environment Department, Social Trends, 1995.)

For example, marriage rates were low in Denmark in 1981 but they had increased by 1992. Religious, cultural and social differences, plus differing legal requirements, account for the rest of the variations.

Since the 1980s, the proportion of lone mothers has stabilized in the UK, but the proportion of single, never married mothers has more than doubled.

The whole ball game is changing. The conventional shape of family life has changed, not just in the UK but right across Europe. Experiences of, and attitudes to, marriage are changing. People are choosing to cohabit before

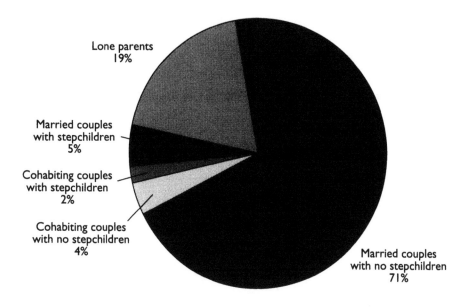

Figure 12 Families with dependent children, by type. (Source: Office of Population Censuses and Surveys, Social Trends, 1995.)

marriage, which has the effect of reducing marriage rates overall and increasing the age at first marriage.

A report written by Labour MP Frank Field, Chairman of the House of Commons Social Security Select Committee, *Making Welfare Work* (published by the Institute of Community Studies, 1995) says that there were 16 million claims for means-tested help in 1993. These included income support, family credit, housing benefits and council tax benefit – 'Safety Net' benefits (Figure 13). When those claiming more than once are removed, the net figure was just under 9.8 million, equivalent to roughly half of all households in the UK. Field argues that the benefits system is 'creaking at the seams'. He says:

Few, except those who abuse it, can make sense of its 25 benefits and six-page means-test application form.

Field makes the point that half the benefit claimants are aged between 19 and 39. A tragedy when you think that this is the time of life when we would expect people to be at their most economically active – laying the foundation for the rest of their lives.

Table 8 Marriage and divorce rates per 1000 population: EC comparisons, 1981 and 1991*

	Marriages		Divorces	
	1981	1992	1981	1992
United Kingdom	7.1	5.4	2.8	3.0
Belgium	6.5	5.8	1.6	2.2
Denmark	5.0	6.2	2.8	2.5
France	5.8	4.7	1.6	1.9
West Germany	5.8	5.6	2.0	1.7
Greece	7.3	4.7	0.7	0.6
Italy	5.6	5.3	0.2	0.5
Luxemburg	5.5	6.4	1.4	1.8
The Netherlands	6.0	6.2	2.0	2.0
Portugal	7.7	7.1	0.7	1.3
Spain	5.4	5.5	0.3	0.7
EC Average	6.0	5.4	1.5	1.6

*Source: Eurostat.

The total cost of all benefits is equal to a contribution of £15 per day from every working taxpayer.

Leaving aside the cost and the increasing numbers of people who claim them, do benefits do what we want them to do? Do they work?

Let me introduce you to Dave, his wife Sandra, and their two kids Jason and Kyle. Dave earns £60 a week working part-time in a factory. With means-tested benefits, the net family income is £125 (after housing costs). This is not much more than Dave would get if he was unemployed and

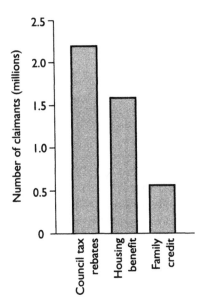

Figure 13 Number of benefit claimants by type of benefit in 1994. Note that child benefit is universal and so is not included. (Source: Field, F (1995) *Making Welfare Work*, Report of the Social Security Select Committee of the House of Commons, Institute of Community Studies.)

stayed in bed all day. But heaven forbid Dave should catch the eye of his boss and get a pay rise. Because of the perverse 'incentives' in the system, means-tested help is reduced as income rises, so if Dave earned another £10 a week, he would have to increase his gross wage to about £140 and earn a total of £200. Where is the incentive?

Perhaps I should remind you that Frank Field is a Labour politician. I felt I should do that before you read what else he has to say. This is not for the faint-hearted!

> The time has come to revolutionize the Welfare State. The system we have penalizes those who work hard and have savings. We don't reward honesty. The time has come to reconstruct welfare. We need to encourage self-interest, self-improvement and altruism once more.

Wait for it, there is more.

> Payment of income support should be linked to a plan for career development.

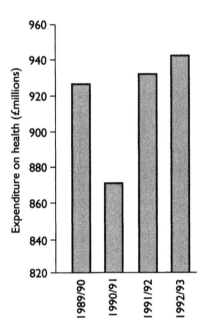

Figure 14 Expenditure on health by the top 400 charities. (Source: Charities Aid Foundation.)

He concludes that smart card technology should be used to help to stamp out fraud, and SAS-style antifraud officers should lead imaginative countermeasures.

Frank Field's view of **Futureproofing** the welfare system is to reinvent it. He wants to see locally elected Welfare Stakeholder Boards, with real power, running the system, a new insurance scheme and the universalization of private pension provision, all run by the boards.

Popular socialism? Certainly, it isn't state capitalism. The fascinating fact, the really intriguing point, is that whatever their politics, thinkers from all sides are coming to the view that what we've got today is no good for tomorrow.

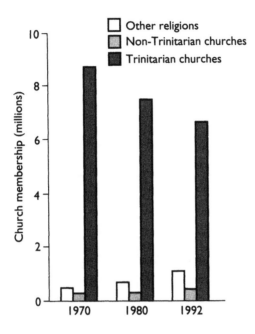

Figure 15 Membership of churches. (Source: Christian Research Association.)

When all else fails

Big players in social welfare are, of course, the charities and churches. The relief of poverty, a Victorian aspiration, is born again. The contributions they make, particularly in the health sector, are notable (Figure 14). But, it's not such good news for the churches. If they were businesses some of them would be broke! Much of the money they invest in schemes, in housing, hostels, direct grants and loans comes from the collection bowl. As Figure 15 shows, fewer people are going to Church and fewer church-goers means less money collected. For how long can the churches continue to play a frontline role?

In 1995, Cardinal Hume, head of the Catholic Church in the UK, announced that a committee would look at the issues of poverty and charity and the role of the Church. Quite what the significance of that move is, who knows? Perhaps he is trying to 'futureproof' the Church!

CHAPTER TWELVE **Pop, goes the weasel!**

But in this world nothing can be said to be certain, except death and taxes
Benjamin Franklin

Put another way, who is going to pay for all this? Technology will rob more people of their jobs than recession ever will, there will be fewer people in the workplace from whom government can harvest taxes. The options are plain: higher taxes or fewer state services, placing greater reliance on the individual.

The options are unattractive. Self-reliance is plainly beyond some citizens. Higher taxes means greater disincentives for people to work hard.

The experiences of the USA and to some extent those of the UK in the Thatcher years, confirm that higher taxes lead to more tax evasion, fiddling and crookery. Lower taxes mean a higher yield for the Treasury.

In the UK, the so-called 'black economy' (money that passes through the economy that is not taxed), is estimated to be worth about £5 bn – one-fifth of the defence budget.

Figure 16 shows the level of taxation in the UK compared with that in other countries.

Since 1979, 1.2 million people in the UK have been taken out of direct taxation altogether. Trumpeted as an achievement by the politicians, it is actually anything but! Why have so many people been taken out of taxation? The sad answer is that they are too poor to pay.

But there is more to taxation than direct taxation. To get the full picture,

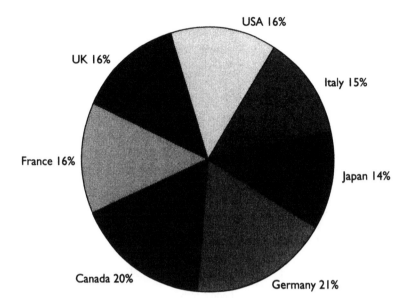

Figure 16 International comparison of direct taxation and social security as a percentage of personal income. (Source: Organization for Economic Co-operation and Development.)

we also need to look at the amount of indirect taxes paid in the UK (Figure 17).

Have you arrived at a conclusion? The poorer you are the more you pay in indirect taxation. The bottom fifth income group pays a higher proportion of income in indirect taxes than the other groups. For homes in the top fifth income group, indirect taxation took 16% of their income, but it accounted for 31% for those in the bottom fifth.

Government's ability to gather taxes is the foundation on which all our public services are based. As fewer people are economically active, either because of retirement or unemployment, so the demand for public services and tax-based benefits increases. There is an inextricable link between employment, social circumstances and health. Greater pressure on public services is inevitable.

For individuals and organizations there are no surprises – more taxes and

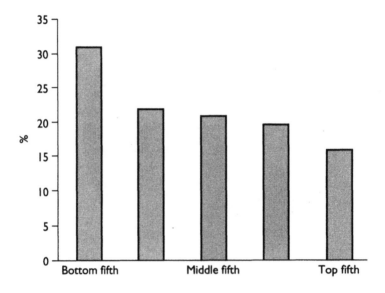

Figure 17 Indirect taxation as a percentage of disposable income, by income groupings, in 1993. (Source: Central Statistical Office.)

greater self-reliance will become a feature of life unless our public services are made to be more effective and efficient. Business-like public services are not popular, and governments need to do popular things to survive. Business-like means reorganization, measurement, comparison, rationalization. Public sector means politics, manoeuvring, compromise and finding a middle course.

Here's something else you should know. The amount spent in the UK on social security benefits is rising (Figure 18). It won't be long before close to £100 million will be spent on welfare benefits alone.

The huge increase in social security spending is not because the value of benefits has risen, it is because the number of people claiming them has shot through the roof. In 1979 there were 7 million claimants; in 1993 there were 11 million.

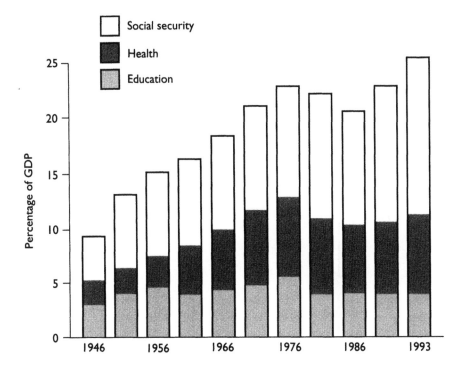

Figure 18 Comparison of welfare and other state expenditure as a proportion of gross domestic product (GDP). (Source: London School of Economics.)

How is the rest of our money spent?

In the years since 1979, spending has increased on social security, health and education. Spending on trade and industry, housing and defence has fallen. The 'peace dividend' has accounted for the small, but significant, shift in defence spending and the huge change in spending on housing is probably accounted for partly by the local authorities moving much responsibility for housing to housing associations and partly by the impact of government controls which prevent local authorities from spending the proceeds of the 'right to buy' movement on building new homes. The fall-off in spending on trade and industry is the result of government's non-interventionist policies in industry.

The percentages spent by the other government departments have remained in the same ranking order – the most significant, social security payments, have stayed at the top of the list and, moreover, appear to be increasing most rapidly.

Figure 19 shows spending on other areas as a percentage of gross domestic product (GDP), comparing 1979 with 1992.

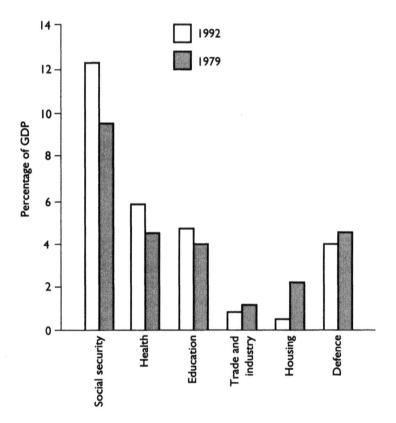

Figure 19 Comparison of state expenditure as a proportion of gross domestic product (GDP) in 1979 and 1992.

CHAPTER THIRTEEN

The non-rules of
Futureproofing

The Golden Rule is that there are no golden rules
George Bernard Shaw

**It's an insane world and in an insane world, sane organizations make no
sense.**
Tom Peters

There is a lot going on, isn't there? One thing is for sure, the future is no
place for the faint-hearted. We have moved into a world where
conventional business approaches make very little sense. Technology and
invention will make today's products and services redundant. Just as we
master the skills we need to survive for today, we will need to learn new
ones for tomorrow.

Old relationships will at best change and most likely go, company
organization will be unrecognizable, and institutions will be shaken to their
foundations. Governments faced with apathy, struggle to keep in touch
with an electorate that is moving away from them.

The average age of the Internet user is 23 years;
you would be pushed to find a politician aged
under 35 years.

A narrowing work base will mean that
governments will have even more trouble
gathering enough money in taxes to meet the
expectations of the very people who will come to
challenge their every motive and move.

'The average
age of the
Internet user
is 23 years;
you would be
pushed to find
a politician
aged under 35
years'

Conventional education will leave us unprepared for the world as it will become, and our values and beliefs will be stretched and challenged.

What will the changes in our society mean for organizations and the people who work in them? More importantly, what can we do to take advantage of these changes?

Wacky ideas for a wacky world

There is a phrase I used to use a lot. It is one of those glib little numbers that trip off the tongue and make people laugh one of those embarrassed laughs that tell me it has struck a chord and is making them think, too. I am not sure where it came from, it is probably a 1970s Americanism.

None of us plan to fail, we simply fail to plan.

It is a phrase born of the time when planning, strategic direction and all that other good stuff was playing a central role in the development of organizations. A range of paper tools, designed to help organizations sort themselves out and grow.

Looking back over the years to the 1970s, it is clear that far from encouraging growth, processes and systems have been more of a corporate straightjacket than a beanpole to grow against.

> 'Looking back over the years to the 1970s, it is clear that far from encouraging growth, processes and systems have been more of a corporate straightjacket than a beanpole to grow against'

In their book *Managing Across Borders* (Harvard Business School Press, Boston, 1989), Chris Bartlett and Sumantra Goshal compare two organizations – Norton (industrial abrasives) and 3M – and their approach to corporate planning. In the 1970s, market strategies and management systems were starting to make an impact on the corporate boardroom, new techniques that measured performance and predicted results.

Norton was committed to state-of-the-art management systems.

Nevertheless, its attempts at diversification were not successful and the results disappointing. In 1990 the company was subsumed by the French firm Compagnie de Saint-Gobain.

3M, on the other hand, placed very little emphasis on top-down management, and focused on encouraging engineers and sales people to come up with good ideas to develop into new products and services. For five years running, 3M was in the *Fortune* magazine's list of Most Admired Corporations.

What makes an organization work? I mean really work, not just survive

In their book *Competing for the Future* (Harvard Business School Press, Boston, 1994), Gary Hamel and C. K. Prahalad ask us to transpose ourselves back a decade or so and make some investment decisions. Play the market, have a punt, and make, or lose, some money.

Would we, they ask, have invested in these companies?

- Volkswagen
- CBS
- Xerox
- RCA
- PanAm
- IBM.

I guess the answer would be 'yes!' We would have been pleased to have shares in any of them. All of them the great international corporations of our time. Strong reputations, in-depth technological back-up and a huge corporate bank account.

Now play the game a different way; this time, make a choice between:

- Volkswagen and Honda

- CBS and CNN
- Xerox and Canon
- RCA and Sony
- PanAm and British Airways
- IBM and Compaq.

Each of these vast organizations has been eclipsed by others that were smaller and came from nowhere. In 1970, when German engineers visited Honda to see what it was up to, they dismissed the Japanese efforts as 'pitiful'. We have RCA to thank for the creation of colour TV. RCA protected its position in the market with intricate patents and design copyright. Sony realized no one makes any money by going to court (except the lawyers) and understood it had to find another way of breaking into the market (reminds you of BT and its ISDN initiative?). So, it simply out-innovated RCA and left it standing.

Ted Turner's CNN was dismissed as 'all show', now it is the world's number one news network station. Canon had dreamed of beating Xerox and did so in the mid-1980s when Canon's production volume made it the world's top copier manufacturer. Incidentally, it pulled the same trick against Leica, the German camera manufacturer.

What energized these companies? The answer is simple: they knew what they wanted, defined it and went for it. British Airways (BA) wanted to be the World's Favourite Airline. It told its staff that's what it wanted and it told its customers. By 1992 it had achieved it.

Now, let's bring Hamel and Prahalad's game up to date:

- Honda or Proton
- British Airways or Virgin Airlines
- Compaq or Tadpole Technology

Korea's Proton car manufacturer looks set to make huge steps forward as it exports not only cars but manufacturing rights. The battle with BA and Virgin has filled pages of newsprint and made many lawyers even richer.

What BA does not seem to realize is that Richard Branson, the Virgin boss, wants to beat BA. He really, deep down, from his boots up, wants to beat BA. His staff know it and his customers know it; the chances are that together they will beat BA.

For two years running, computer Whiz-kids Tadpole Technology has been at the top of the list of firms ranked by the percentage of sales revenue that is spent on research and development (R&D). The top five are shown in Table 9.

Table 9 Companies ranked by percentage of sales revenue spent on R&D

1995 (1994)			Total 4 year sales (£m)	Total 4 year added value (£m) (£m)	Total 4 year R&D expenditure	R&D as % of added value
1	(1)	Tadpole Technology	77.45	18.31	7.60	41.5
2	–	Telspec	59.96	22.46	6.41	28.5
3	–	Gresham Telecomputing	25.88	11.79	3.31	28.1
4	(5)	Wellcome	8070.90	4754.60	1263.50	26.6
5	–	Zeneca	16158.00	6368.00	1677.00	26.3
		Industry average of top 50 companies	213285.75	91285.97	15169.28	16.6

*Source: VI Consultants/IOD 1995.

What makes these companies do so well? Successful organizations do two things really well; two things that mark them out as different: they involve their staff and are fanatical about communications.

The department of damned good ideas

Preparing an organization for the future is as much about making it fast, proactive and energetic as it is about anything else, and that means tapping into the skills and talents of the people who work there.

When people come to work they leave behind a household they are perfectly able to run and budget for. They leave behind their ability to plan their holidays, run a youth club, lay out a garden, undertake DIY projects and manage their relationships. They leave at home their talent for bargain-hunting and buying complicated products like life assurance, new cars, mortgages and computers. When they come to work they are underutilized and wasted; 90% of what they are competent at never gets used at work. People can usually do more, accomplish more and make a far bigger contribution than we give them credit for.

At the beginning of the reform of the NHS, hospital trusts were set up – self-governing with their own board of directors and responsible for their own strategic direction. The trusts, formerly the hospital units, were beset with problems. 'Spanish' practices were rife and the organizations worked in administrative slums. The Homewood Trust, in Chertsey, Surrey, was no different from anywhere else. I was appointed chairman of the Homewood in 1991.

The problems were overwhelming. Bereft of answers, the board decided to ask the one group of people most likely to have the answers, the staff, what should be done.

> 'When they come to work they are underutilized and wasted; 90% of what they are competent at never gets used at work. People can usually do more, accomplish more and make a far bigger contribution then we give them credit for'

Homewood embarked on the 'Help Team' approach. Help Teams were composed of staff volunteers, volunteers that came from across the organization regardless of length of service or seniority. All they had to have to qualify for membership of the team was a genuine interest in the problem. When something came up the board used the internal newspaper, but more often the grapevine, to ask for people to come forward and help.

The Help Teams were resourced with secretarial support and had free access to any part of the organization in pursuit of a solution to a problem or task. Critics of the approach predicted the staff would recommend high priced answers that would be impossible to implement and the whole approach would raise expectations that could not be met. The staff would go away disillusioned and morale would fall.

In practice, the experience was quite to the contrary. The staff used their powers with care and respect, their ideas were fresh and always deliverable. Indeed, the quality of the decisions made by the Help Teams was always better and more innovative than decisions that the Board or a manager could have arrived at in isolation.

It worked, and it worked well. Thorny issues that the board had not dared to grasp were handled by the teams. Overtime, which was costing the organization a fortune, was banned in favour of full staffing and an internal agency arrangement established to cover unplanned absences. The use of external agency staff was ended.

Staff housing allocation, always a minefield of problems, was settled by a Help Team, as was staff safety and security policy, environmental policy, child care facilities and a host of other issues, all sorted and settled by the people who knew most about the problems.

> 'The staff used their powers with care and respect, their ideas were fresh and always deliverable. Indeed, the quality of the decisions made by the Help Teams was always better and more innovative than decisions that the board or a manager could have arrived at in isolation'

Anita Roddick's Body Shop has a similar approach. She calls it the Department of Damned Good Ideas.

The future is in Littlehampton

Don't worry about getting an MBA, get a ticket to the future and all the education you will need for just £4.80. Invest in yourself, and for just under a fiver you can go on a trip to Roddick's Body Shop empire at Littlehampton.

To be frank the last thing I wanted to do was to be dragged through a women's perfume and bottled jollop factory. But boy, am I glad I went! Go and see for yourself how a company should be run. You can feel the excitement in the air. Talk to the staff and feel their commitment. They all know why they are there (no, not merely to earn a wage), they all understand the mission of the company, why it is in business and where it is going.

The scribblers in the City and on Wall Street have given the Body Shop a bad time. It's easy to see why. Here is an odd-ball company doing odd-ball things and making a success in a very competitive market. Body Shop knows it cannot last for ever, as it is. 'As it is', that's the important bit. Because they are flexible, because they are unconventional and because they know their trading environment is changing (like the 14-year-olds do), Body Shop will transform and Body Shop will survive, I have no doubt. They are **Futureproofed**.

Go and see the future in Littlehampton, and if you don't come away with a good idea for your organization – leave, because you've lost it!

Reading it in the eyes

If they haven't heard it, you haven't said it.
Harvey Thomas – pinched from Marshall MacClure!

Organizations I talk to about communications usually tell me they have got communications sewn up. We have a newsletter, they say. Send out a newsletter, tell people what's going on and that's the end of it. Wrong! There is much more to it than that. Communications is not a management bugle, sounded from the top of the 51st floor. Communications are what makes some companies different from the rest.

Reinventing communications

The new definition of corporate communications concerns the management of information flows; real information about how the company is doing, budget information, policy; controlling the organization through information management and communications; communications in a supporting management role; communications that become a system in themselves, helping managers to manage themselves as well as the business; communications that harness ambition and disengage from control.

There is a furnishing store, represented in over 15 countries and with a sales turnover of US$5 billion, that does not have a budgeting system – it was dumped in 1992. That company is Sweden's Ikea.

Ikea controls the costs of 10 000 product lines sold in 100 stores worldwide and purchased from nearly 200 suppliers in a very competitive environment.

'There is a furnishing store, represented in over 15 countries and with a sales turnover of US$5 billion, that does not have a budgeting system – it was dumped in 1992'

Ikea manages with a set of ratios that are communicated around the company, giving all staff real-time access to up to date data. The ratios are set up to create competition between departments and managers. Now that is what I call communication: communication that does more than empower staff; this type of communication engages people in the running of the business.

Redefined communications allow us to open the corporate store cupboard, distribute the information in there and use it to competitive advantage. You see, information is not knowledge. Information only becomes knowledge when it is passed on, and at that point knowledge becomes power.

Back to one of my favourite businesses, the Body Shop. It has more than 700 shops in 40 countries. In each one you will find a video recorder and a fax machine. Anita Roddick uses them to saturate her staff with messages and information. She goes further. She visits her stores holds regular meetings, sometimes at her home, with staff of all grades and seniority in the organization. This is the hallmark of leadership, and is what marks out some companies from the rest. There is no substitute for the staff hearing it first from the boss. Good news, bad news or just an update of some old news, it comes best, as Ingvar Kamprad, founder of Ikea, would say: 'mouth to ear'.

I have lost count of the number of times I have wandered into an organization and been depressed by the noticeboard. Management by memorandum is not what staff want. A new memo pinned to a noticeboard does not excite much interest. If staff have to read news they would rather read it in the eyes of the boss than on a piece of paper.

'If staff have to read news they would rather read it in the eyes of the boss than on a piece of paper'

Next time you fly Virgin, don't be surprised if Richard Branson is serving the drinks. He regularly turns up, talks to the staff and the customers, and learns more about his airline business.

Information technology is life or death and nothing in between

For many business leaders born of a gas lamp generation, the management of information by the use of technology is a bewildering jungle. Technology is fashion, and it is fashionable to disown technology. You must have heard the words: 'Oh, we have computers and the like but I leave it to the whiz-kids to sort out.' Dangerous effete-ism. Press F10 and exit this company.

'On switching to computer-driven business, the company's customer satisfaction rating jumped from 55% to over 90%'

Nick Kingsbury, is managing director of G Kingsbury, a company that has its roots in the nineteenth century. The company is in the vehicle hire, service and sales business. Kingsbury admits he knew nothing about computers and, until 1993, maintained manual systems for the whole of his accounting and management systems.

On switching to computer-driven business, the company's customer satisfaction rating jumped from 55% to over 90%. The information available on the computer system enabled reception staff to advise customers on the progress of their vehicles through the workshops and enabled staff to participate in quality improvement clinics based on real-time information.

The company took a high risk approach to the installation of computerized systems. It was introduced at the beginning of a new financial year and the old manual system was dropped. Kingsbury argues that the approach galvanized team spirit. The system had to work, and work it did. Following computerization, profitability jumped from £200 000 to £300 000.

Kingsbury says: 'I used to liken the place to Fawlty Towers. Now I have kicked the habit of living in the past.'

CHAPTER FOURTEEN

Change – what change?

You should never have your best trousers on when you turn out to fight for
freedom and truth.
Ibsen

In the spring of 1994, I was talking with a group of managers who work in
the NHS. They told me their lives were impossible. They were at their
wits'-end, pressured beyond endurance. There was no way they could do
their jobs. They could not 'manage', they told me, as the goal posts kept
being moved. I've heard that one before. The trouble was, *they* believed it.
'Everything keeps changing,' they complained, 'how are we supposed to
manage? No one can manage in that environment.'

Frankly, I didn't know whether to laugh or cry.
They didn't like the answer I gave them. They
were not pleased with me when I pointed out
that without change there would be no need for
managers. Without change we could get along
with administrators, and the wages bill would be a
lot cheaper. Change is what management exists
for.

'Without change we could get along with administrators, and the wages bill would be a lot cheaper. Change is what management exists for'

Things are supposed to change, they are at least
supposed to get better. But most times things
seem to get worse! Things will get thrown into the
air, turned upside down, trashed, binned and
scrapped. If you don't do it someone else will. If
your organization, your company isn't in the
process of change, you can bet your competitors
are. Change is fundamental to competition.

A horse can win a race by a short head. Thousands if not millions of pounds ride on the winner and a short head is enough, just a few inches. The 60 yard dash, the electrifying short sprint in indoor athletics, separates the winners and losers by milliseconds. That's all it takes to win: a short head or a millisecond. Tough to win, easy to lose. Competing for market share, competing to hang on to what you've got, competition and change go hand in hand.

The 14 year olds are looking at how 'change influences business behaviour' in their GCSE syllabus. Ross Ashby wrote about it as long ago as 1958. The 14 year olds will find out what Ashby knew nearly 40 years ago, that the pressure to change organizations, to reflect and respond to the environment in which they operate, will move from a once-in-a-lifetime review or a new product cycle every 10 years, to now, this afternoon.

Change won't confine itself neatly, concurrently, to the annual strategy cycle. The pressure is on and we will be forced into reassessing daily what we are doing. Change becomes a way of life, change is the norm. If we've got to worry about change, the game is up. We must move past change.

> 'Change won't confine itself neatly, concurrently, to the annual strategy cycle'

Change is the one thing guaranteed to get everyone going. People get uptight, they feel threatened, behave defensively and fly off the handle. Organizations that are unprepared for the pace of change will be caught unawares.
Organizations must be groomed to expect change, encouraged to expect it, trained to respond to it, get excited by it.

Smart change

Change is not a simple one-way street. You want change, drive it into the organization. Change something overnight? Easy, but how many people will it affect? Change is inevitably about getting better performance. You don't get better performance by screwing people up, getting them uptight, making them feel threatened, behave defensively and fly off the handle.

Make change the norm, unexceptional, average. If you are a manager, owner or leader of an organization, review what you do and stop talking change, talk smart change. Speak the language of doing it differently, improving a service, revamping, be smart about the language of change. Would you rather be on the receiving end of change or in the vanguard of helping to do something differently in the customer's interest?

The four rules of smart change

Everyone is a winner

Oh yes they are! Everyone *is* a winner – if you'll let them be. People want to do a good job. Many don't do a good job and the reason is that no one lets them. People want to do a great job. They want to go home feeling they have achieved something and they want to go home looking forward to coming back for some more tomorrow. The reason people don't do a good job is that managers and organizations won't let them. We fence in talent, build boundaries around bright people, lock up genius, stamp on initiative and snuff out instinct.

Look, here's an example of what I mean. A customer turns up in an organization somewhere (it doesn't matter which one or where, it's probably your place!), bitching like hell over something or other.

> **'Organizations that put their customers first, put hierarchies last'**

The frontliner ducks the flack, makes a note and passes it up the line. The supervisor knows there's nothing she can do about it and passes it to the manager. The manager passes it to production and production shifts it over to packaging. Packaging notifies shipping, and shipping tells sales. The sales manager sends a memo to the area sales manager and the area sales manager phones the sales rep and tells him to go and see the customer and find out what it was all about. Assuming the customer is not by now at the lawyers or the undertakers, the sales rep will turn up, get his ears bitten off, and go home and shout at his wife because 'he's having a bad day'.

Don't bother to count – there are 10 people in the chain.

What could have happened, is that the frontliner could have found out what was wrong and fixed it. Could the frontliner have been the supervisor, manager, production, packaging, shipping, the sales manager, the area sales manager and the sales rep? Yes. Absolutely. Why not? Empowered by the magic of a displeased customer, benighted by an upset punter, you bet the frontliner can be anybody he or she needs to be to be able to send the customer home with a smile. Job fixed, on the spot. It can be done. Organizations that put their customers first, put hierarchies last.

The customer is not interested in who the supervisor or manager is, or who does production, packaging, shipping, or what the name of the sales manager is, or the fact that the area sales manager and the sales rep are Martians. The customer wants it fixed, sorted and out of the way.

If people think they can; they will

The simple act of knowing what is expected of them and agreeing to it makes people better performers. You can, if you think you can. Expectations, personal, departmental, corporate, whatever, are driven by goals. Marching in step, keeping in tune, call it what you like – share the vision, share the work and share the success.

'You can, if you think you can'

Organizations that have a corporate vision have nothing if the vision isn't shared, known and understood by everybody who works in that organization and comes into contact with it.

Peter Drucker, American management guru, describes three people working on a building site. They were all doing the same job and were asked the same question: 'What are you doing?' One answered, 'breaking rocks', another said, 'earning a living', the third replied, 'helping to build a cathedral'. Share the vision and you get a better organization.

In their book *The Strategic Management Blue Print* (Blackwell Business Press, Oxford, 1993), Paul Dobson and Ken Starkey conclude that mission is:

... a definition of the long term vision of the organization ...

Sorry guys, I don't agree. Mission is not just identifying the long-term aims of the organization. Mission is what people try and deliver every day when they come to work.

Mission is what shades, colours and gives texture to our contact with customers and the people we provide our services for. Mission is how we choose our suppliers, how we engage our staff and how we live in our environment. The vision, the mission, is corporate strategy, nothing more is needed.

Share it with your people. Write it on the wall, print it on every piece of corporate stationery, on the security passes that your people wear clipped to their lapels, on your products, on the serviettes in the canteen and on a sticker on every telephone.

Learning is a continuum, not an end

If we are wise, we never leave school. Remember the German apprentices whose skills are redundant by the time they get to use them (see page 52)? The problem is not just what we learn, it is also where we learn.

It really cannot be long before the great universities realize that running a campus, providing all those 'rooms' for their students, all those canteens and sporting facilities, all those lecture halls, that great pile of bricks, is a mug's game. Somebody bright is going to discover that lectures can be sent up on to the Astra satellite to be downloaded in the middle of the night, on to the videos of students all over Europe for a fraction of what it costs to heat, light, insure, and paint a pile of bricks. And the students will be sleeping in their own beds, eating their mum's cooking and using their local sports centre.

> 'It really cannot be long before the great universities realize that running a campus, providing all those 'rooms' for their students, all those canteens and sporting facilities, all those lecture halls, that great pile of bricks, is a mug's game'

If the student needs access to the library, the whole lot will be on CD-ROM. The Internet will have the university bulletin board, and work will be done at home, on-screen and E-mailed to the tutor (in a cottage in the Cotswolds) for marking and comment. The tutors will love it – no more rotten handwriting to decipher! The invisible campus, student-free but packed with people discovering, finding out and learning. The time taken to achieve a degree will be halved or extended to a lifetime – it will be up to you.

Lifetime learning. A lifetime spent hunting down and capturing new knowledge and releasing it when we've done with it. No, I'm not crazy (not yet), think about those German apprentices. I don't believe they are the only ones running up the down escalator of learning. The doctors in the British NHS come close – 14 years to become a consultant.

> 'A lifetime spent hunting down and capturing new knowledge and releasing it when we've done with it'

Unipart, the British car accessory and parts manufacturer, has turned itself into a university. The director of finance is the head of the maths faculty, and the head of information technology is the head of the university's IT department, transferring skills around the organization.

Sorry to do this to you, but Anita's done it too. Back to Littlehampton, where Anita Roddick's Body Shop factory is a learning organization with a purpose. Staff are given tokens to 'trade' for learning. Someone in sales wants to learn about budgeting and he trades tokens with someone in the finance department. Need to know how to get the best out of your software? Trade tokens with the IT people or someone who is better at it than you are. Collect the tokens, cash them in and use them to learn new things outside the organization.

Learning what you want when its needed. Learning – no big deal.

The customer is the boss

If you think the customer is King you are wrong. The customer is the Dictator.
Lord Seif, Marks & Spencer

I love the story about the priest in a small Irish town. He is sitting at his desk, writing his sermon for Sunday, when he looks out over the fields and sees a man walking towards him. The priest can hardly believe his eyes. The man has long flowing hair and a beard. He is wearing a white robe. As he walks, a shaft of light follows him. He is surrounded by angels.

The priest reaches for the telephone and rings the Vatican. He tells his story and is put through to the Pope. 'Holy Father,' says the priest, 'what shall I do?'

The voice at the other end of the 'phone answers: 'Look busy it could be the boss!'

King, dictator, boss. The customer is all of these things.

Small businesses are better at looking after customers than big businesses. Fact. They are closer to the customer. Small businesses are building a business, they achieve more by giving their customers what they want. Pensioners can't buy three eggs in a prepackaged-obsessed supermarket, they can in the corner shop.

Solution to the customer problem – make all organizations small organizations. They may form part of a bigger whole, make them federal, but make them free. Free to focus on the customer, put the customer in the spotlight.

Richard Branson has just the quote we're looking for.

Once it gets impersonal, it's time to break the company up.

The organization reflects what the people at the top are, do and believe

Here is a list of what I believe.

- Top people in the organization must demonstrate that they are genuinely interested in the organization. Being visible in the organization helps to demonstrate that interest; being invisible does not.

- Most successful companies are fanatical about keeping in touch with the business.

- The organization must measure itself against a handful of fundamental criteria (mission and values). That is the zero base. Zero basing – reviewing the base – is a constant process that must become second nature to the organization.

- Successful organizations extract far more from their staff by way of commitment than do average companies. Invariably that commitment comes from the example of the people at the top. The more the boss does, the more the staff will do.

- Get the organization right, and look after the staff as a result of having a successful organization.

- Successful organizations have a continuous interest in innovation and the process of change.

- Leaders are visible, they have a clear vision, which they believe in passionately and incite others to subscribe to. They thrive where people have clear objectives.

- Employee confidence that top people in the organization know what they are doing is best derived from face to face encounters.

- I am less interested in corporate organization than I am in corporate culture.

- Leaders are active, rather than reactive.

- What else is there but winning?

What do you believe? Write it down now.

The Secret Pages
The things you'll never learn on an
MBA course

CHAPTER FIFTEEN

Recognize this place?

There needs to be a constant recognition that you have to jump out of existing structures in order to let new business in
Who said that? Read on and find out ...

Draw an organizational chart of your place. Does it look anything like this?

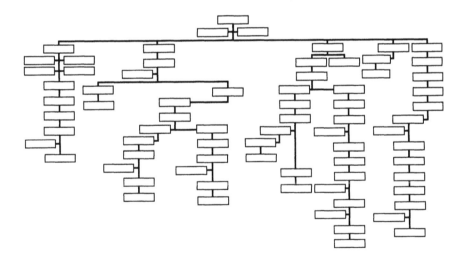

Figure 20 Your place?

Spot the ball

I guess you know where the boss fits and I'm pretty sure, if you're not the boss, you will know where you are. But, I have a question for you. There is some one I want you to plot on the chart – position them. Just a simple cross will do. You don't even have to know their name.

Ready, got your pen in hand? OK, indicate on the chart the precise position of the customer. Yes, you remember, the customer, the service user, the punter, the person who pays for it all. Where do they go?

Spot the ball competitions are easier … and more rewarding!

North and south people

Assuming the 'boss' is 'north' and the rest of us are 'south' and accepting that customer contact is usually with 'south' people, how many levels does a north person have to abseil down to get near a south person and a customer? How long does it take to get a decision made and who makes the decisions anyway? How do people communicate with each other and how many copies of a memo do they have to generate?

On the example chart, which is taken from a real, live chart, (the names have been removed to protect the innocent), the answer is thirteen. Now, I can't tell you the name of the organization that I have pinched this chart from (because the NHS gets very upset), but I can promise you it's the real thing.

Perhaps a more telling question is; how many levels has a south person, or a service user, got to scale before they can get to the north people?

North people are seldom aware of the problem. I have spoken at lots of conferences and in countless boardrooms about this issue. A classic (and what would be a hysterically funny anecdote if it wasn't so serious) concerns a district council in the south of England.

I challenged a Council chief executive on the shape of his organization. He said he would take on board what I had said and come up with some ideas for my consideration.

A week later he wrote to me enclosing a copy of his new organizational chart.

Here it is:

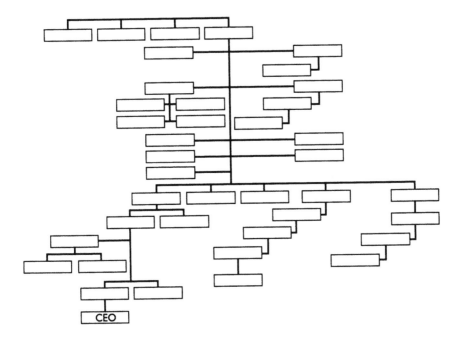

Figure 21 The new organizational chart.

He was very proud of the fact that he had flipped the chart upside down and shown himself at the bottom of the chart, in order, as he put it, 'to reflect the contribution of his hard working staff'.

No, no, no boss, you've missed the point! Turning the chart upside down, changing north people into south people is not the answer. The point is, where is the customer.

He had another go and produced this:

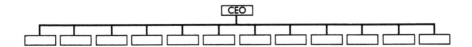

Figure 22 Who are you trying to kid?

Ho, ho, nice try – who are you trying to kid. All those cute little boxes are departments that are like buds on a tree in springtime; waiting to burst into more little boxes. Although it is true, a flat structure is better, I call this one the 'last supper' model. Try getting the salt passed from east to west and you'll see the communications difficulty.

I am not specially in favour of wasting a lot of time in pursuit of the ideal organizational structure. My real belief is that it should be the shape of the customer. However, if pushed, in the broadest of terms, let's dump the 'name on the box' approach – this is a shape I do like.

Dunkin'-doughnuts

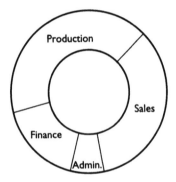

Figure 23 Dunkin'-doughnut.

Now put a cross where the customer might be. The customer can be anywhere on the chart. Inside or outside the ring, accessing, directly that bit of the service they need to interface with. They dip in or dip out at any point – dunkin' into the organization.

The best examples of this type of approach to structure I have found are in the newborn insurance-by-telephone companies. Call them for a quotation or a query and a recorded voice (no expensive 'Hello Girls'), gives a range of options and departments for you to access by touch-tone telephone. The menu of choice is further subdivided, giving more options and in moments you are speaking to the person you really want to deal with. Quotes, claims, payments, queries, press the number and you are straight into the organization. Unlike old style insurance companies where you could be shunted around departments for ages, repeating your name a thousand times and still not getting what you want. Direct access, lower overheads and cheaper premiums.

Inside the ring or anywhere outside – and you can do this:

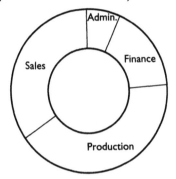

Figure 24 Spin the organization around.

Spin the organization around to line up with the position of the customer – provide the correct customer interface.

Or this:

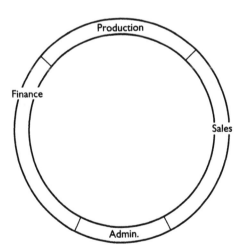

Figure 25 Very thin dunkin'-doughnut!

Very thin – yes I like this one!

A pain in the back

A couple of years ago I did what most middle-aged men shouldn't do and played squash! I collapsed in a sweaty, plump heap and ended up with a damaged disk in my back, requiring an operation to put right. Following the surgery were two wonderful years of pain free living that gave way to the sinister re-emergence of the symptoms. A long term painkiller and anti-inflammatory treatment was required – called an epidural. An injection into the offending area. Minor day-case stuff, with an anaesthetic.

On the appointed day, early in the morning, I showed up at the hospital. The ward clerk made a note of my name and address and I waited. The anesthetist turned up and made a note of my name and address, took my blood pressure and asked me if I was asthmatic or had any allergies.

Next, the house-man (junior doctor) turned up and made a note of my name and address, took my blood pressure and asked me if I was asthmatic or had any allergies.

He was followed by the senior registrar on the surgeon's team who made a note of my name and address, took my blood pressure and asked me if I was asthmatic or had any allergies.

The ward Sister followed who announced there was no bed for me as they had been 'very busy' and I would have to be transferred to another ward. I was met at my new ward by the Sister who said they were not sure if I could be admitted as they had run out of clean sheets and were waiting for the laundry to 'send up fresh supplies' and as they 'didn't do this until 10am and the surgeon's list started at 9am I may not get admitted in time'!

After offering to go home and get some clean sheets from my airing cupboard (Oh, they didn't like that idea!), sheets were found and I was admitted by a very sour-faced nursing Sister who made a note of my name and address, took my blood pressure and asked me if I was asthmatic or had any allergies.

Finally the great man attended upon me. The surgeon popped in. He said he wouldn't trouble me with all the paperwork but: he took my blood pressure and asked me if I was asthmatic or had any allergies.

There is something expensively, irritatingly, fundamentally, gobsmackingly wrong with the organizational structure of that hospital. An admissions assistant could have saved the work of five people. Saved not just work but time and money, never mind the frustration. Had it not been the NHS and therefore, I had no choice, I would have taken my business elsewhere. As the internal market, now very much a feature of the modern NHS, starts to take effect, hopefully, these costly practices will be swept aside. Competition between hospitals will force them to become more efficient.

Futureproofed organizations organize around the needs of the customer. They change shape, they are chameleons and they are Plasticine.

It is easy to poke fun at the NHS, but what is it like over at your place?

Call-up

Suggestion. Leave your office, go to the nearest phone box and call yourself up. See how easy you are to get through to. I once suggested this to the chairman of a public company. He took me up on the challenge.

He was furious to find that when he asked for himself by name the switchboard told him 'no one by that name worked there', how right they were!

Mark McCormick, founder of the International Management Group (IMG), said, in 1984 (!),

> The fluidity of business is simply too fast and too formless for existing systems and structures to hold it. Once our structures were in place, we began the ongoing process of ignoring them. I believe this is one of the greatest challenges to almost any established company – a constant recognition that you have to jump out of existing structures in order to let new business in.

I love that quote. Remember, he made it ten years ago! Before the boom in technology, before the Internet, before, mobile 'phones were common place – before the customer revolution that puts who pays for the service at the 'north end' of the business.

I also love the McCormickism: '...a constant recognition that you have to jump out of existing structures in order to let new business in.'

'Jump out, to let in'. I love the concept, 'letting in new business'. Throwing over baggage to take on cargo. Organizations create structures that are barriers and barriers keep out customers and talent.

Thank you Mark, I couldn't have put it better myself! And, I know you have a secret. You spend 90% of your time on doing business and 10% of your time on organization.

Futureproofing lesson; dump structures, regularly!

Who do you have to be?

Has it ever occurred to you that the best companies are run by unconventional people? Whenever you read about the leader of an organization who has done well and achieved success, they have always broken a rule, kicked over the wall of convention or broken a barrier. They have given unlikely people a chance to shine, they have encouraged independence and the cult of the individual. Is it flair? Is it in the genes? Are you born with it? or Can you learn it?

A **Futureproofer** is unconventional. To survive in the world that is on the horizon it is not enough to look for opportunities, you must create them. A **Futureproofer** is four people

> Danny Kaye
> Henry Kissinger
> The Pope
> Christiaan Barnard

...all rolled into one.

Danny Kaye

If you started reading this book at the beginning you will know about my great age! I am old enough to remember 'Uncle Mac'. Uncle Mac was a radio presenter who, on Saturday mornings on the BBC Light Programme (I never thought I would be old enough to reminisce!), presented 'Children's Favourites'. Kids, or their parents, would write in and request a record. The all time, favourite, most played record was Danny Kay performing Hans Christian Andersen's 'The Kings New Clothes'.

I know the words off by heart! The story is about an arrogant King who knew it all. One day a couple of sharp sales types turn up at the palace and sold him a new suit of clothes. They told the King the suit was invisible to fools and could only be seen by wise men. In fact they sold the King a coat hanger! The King is too into himself to realize he had been done. With a flourish the King put on the 'new suit' and paraded himself down the high street. Dutiful subjects are arranged on the pavement to cheer the King and admire the new suit.

They chant suitably admiring chants, with the exception of a small boy, unfazed by events who asks 'why is the King walking down the high street, naked?'

I guess you could argue I took on board my first management lesson at the age of four! The lesson was; don't get swept along by events, don't follow the herd and always ask the question that everyone else is too bashful, (or afraid), to ask.

Challenge conventional wisdom and don't be shy about it. Where would the thousands of companies, who were riding high in the early 1980s, be now, if someone on their boards had made the point: 'It's OK to expand on borrowed money, but what happens if interest rates go up? Can we handle our interest debt payments?' I guess a lot more of them would be around now – employing people and creating wealth.

What would have happened to 'names' at Lloyds, if someone had asked the question: 'How are we fixed if we have a whole string of disasters on the trot?'

Challenging convention and asking the awkward question is never a way to become popular but it is a way to **Futureproof** a lot of what we do.

Henry Kissinger

Henry Alfred Kissinger was sworn in on 22 September 1973 as the fifty-sixth US Secretary of State, a position he held until January 20, 1977. In 1973 he received the Nobel Peace Prize; in 1977 the presidential Medal of Freedom; and in 1986 the Medal of Liberty.

Kissinger was born in Fürth in Germany, moved to the US in 1938, becoming a US citizen in 1943. In 1950 he graduated from Harvard and four years later became a member of the faculty at the University. He has an astonishing life story and his book; *Diplomacy*, Simon & Schuster 1994, is a dense but enlightening read.

The complexities of the problems he dealt with are not for this book. However, the man in the street will, forever, link Kissinger, with 'shuttle diplomacy'. During his 'shuttling' period I was doing business with the US. For many US companies exporting was; 'making something in California and shipping it to Washington'. At a time when America had little influence in the world and lived in a foreign-policy vacuum, the combination of Richard Nixon and Henry Kissinger was formidable, pivotal and changed the US forever.

The phrase 'shuttle diplomacy' was an invention of the newspaper fraternity, to describe a process it had no words for. Kissinger shuttled from one problem to the next, from one protagonist to another, from one side to the other, in a gruelling round of meetings, travels and negotiations. The journalists of the day failed to find a word for the process and invented one! Years later Tom Peters had no such problem; he called it 'management by walking about'.

That's the key. Getting out and about. Finding out, on the ground, what's going on, on the ground, talking to people and solving problems face to face. Forget the memos, shred the status reports, bin the analysis. Go and find out. Roddick turns up at her shops; Branson serves drinks on his aeroplanes; the MD of M&S makes unannounced visits to suppliers; Rocco

Forte spends three nights a week staying in his hotels. Unconventional people do unconventional things and achieve unconventional successes.

In the early days of my time as the Chairman of a hospital Trust, determined to make managers more aware of what was going on in the organization, I conspired with the cleaning staff and locked some managers out of their offices for two days! They worked out of their brief cases, had meetings where the problems were, talked directly to staff and returned 'phone calls on the hoof. The place was never run so well as it was for those two days! It changed the culture of the organization for ever.

Clive Stone owns Redcliffe Catering. He used to work for someone else, saw his opportunity, put his house, his family and his security on the line. Now he runs one of the most successful businesses I have come across. A new-age business.

His staff say he is mad, eccentric, difficult, demanding, annoying and they would die for him. Why? Because he is mad about the business and is always there; eccentric in the way in which he treats his staff – like they are one of the family; difficult to please because he only wants the best, he is a perfectionist; demanding of himself and everyone around him; insisting they discover what a customer really wants and then delivering it; annoying because he turns up to find out what really happens and endlessly changes things around. And he would die for his staff – he says they *are* the business.

Futureproofed organizations are owned, run and staffed by people who are out from behind their desks and into the business, unconventional is their norm.

The Pope

The ability to delegate is the single discriminator between good management and bad. The issue is not about passing work down, it is about building people up. How will we know about the talents of the workforce and our colleagues if we never give them a try? Delegate the tasks you like doing the most – why should you have all the fun? Share the work you least like doing – don't dump it.

Futureproofers delegate to educate.

When you hire people, make it a rule, a golden rule, always, without fail, to hire people who are brighter than you are and let them get on with the job. When the organization is full of the brightest and the best, sell the organization to customers, users, the public and other companies as the place where the bright people are and the place where the job gets done the best – that's your job!

And – when these bright people screw up (and they will), make sure they work in an atmosphere where they can confess without recrimination. British Airways has a senior captain available to listen to flight crews who may have made a mistake during a flight. No recriminations, just learning from each other's experiences and mistakes. Be the Pope – listen to confessions and forgive. If success was easy, everyone would be successful – it is not and they are not. Encourage people who have made mistakes. If you never do anything you can't make a mistake. The future is only for the people who *do* things.

Futureproofed organizations hire the best, take risks, screw-up and learn from the experience. As our environment gets more complex the opportunity for mistakes, misjudgements and missing out gets greater. Recognize it and learn from it.

Christiaan Barnard

On 3 December 1967 the world suddenly found out where Groote Schuur was. It was introduced to the grocer Louis Washkansky and forgot about the 25-year-old bank clerk, Denise Darvall.

Denise was injured in a road accident and was dying. She agreed that her heart could be used in the world's first experiment, to transplant a heart from one human to another. Her kidneys were to be transplanted into a coloured boy in another hospital. History does not seem to have recorded the name of the 'coloured' boy – this was South Africa in the mid-60s. Louis was suffering grave heart failure and Groote Schuur was the hospital where one Christiaan N Barnard, Professor of Cardio-thoracic Surgery had been dreaming of the impossible. To take Denise's heart and transplant it into Louis's chest.

Barnard did it, somehow, against all the odds. The world sat on the edge of its seat and listened to the unfolding story of the first heart transplant. Performed, not in the US or one of London's great teaching hospitals, but in South Africa. In the Groote Schuur Hospital – Afrikaans for 'big shed hospital'! Where was that?

The world gossiped about the news bulletins and the pundits discussed the ethics of man playing God. The thirty doctors and nurses in Barnard's team worried about the new science of tissue rejection.

Christiaan Barnard 'futureproofed' the lives of thousands, if not millions of people. Barnard also teaches us the lessons of vision, determination and debunking the establishment. He decided what he wanted to do and did it. With a background in the NHS you can imagine I have spoken a lot about Professor Barnard. Several times doctors have approached me with their version of the 'inside' story. Apparently a hospital in the UK was on the verge of doing the same thing. Somewhere in the US, 'somebody' was just about to do the same. Always the stories are about 'nearly', 'just', 'almost'. Barnard did it, in the 'big shed'.

Futureproofers get on with the job.

*So, what does it take to be a **Futureproofer**?*

- Ask the questions no one else asks.
- Go and see for yourself what is happening.
- Encourage people to make mistakes.
- Define your vision and JGDI (just go do it).

Is that enough?

Straight answer is – no!

The best present I ever had was a Swiss Army knife. I was the envy of my friends and there wasn't a horse within five miles of where I lived that had a stone left in its hoof!

The knife had a saw, tweezers, pliers, a screwdriver, a magnifying glass, a hoof-pick, an awl and, oh yes, a scalped, sharp knife or two. The knife was a resource centre – and so must you be.

The job market is going to get tougher and more competitive – only the best people will survive. You need to be more than 'just good' at what you do. What am I saying? Expert is not enough? Heavens no! Pick up any commercial directory, any local newspaper, any *Yellow Pages*, any *Thomson Directory* and you will find a thousand, a hundred thousand, millions of people who are experts and can do things ten thousand times better than you. You can't hope to compete. Out-source everything you can. I'm talking about the new specialist, the personal specialist, the resource centre. The indefinable something that makes managers worth 'sleeping on the streets' for. (Remember?)

I'm talking about the **Futureproofed** person who is rounded, informed and different. I started this book with a question – how old are you? – as we move towards the final pages, let me ask you some more questions.

- What newspapers do you read?
- What magazines do you read?
- What TV news programmes do you watch?
- When did you last learn something?
- Can you type?
- Do computers frighten you, or excite you?
- How many holidays do you take?
- What do you do on holiday?

There are no right answers so don't worry!

What newspapers do you read?

Don't bother with any of them! Well, OK, that is over the top. Read a paper for entertainment. Use E-mail to get the news. Real-time, hot news, straight off the wire services Reuters or Press Association. News – raw, as it happens; news without opinion. News that you can make your own mind up about. Try to read a 'foreign' newspaper. *The European* will do, or the *Wall Street Journal*, or the *International Herald Tribune*, or a foreign-language newspaper if you are smart.

Find out what 'outsiders' think of what is happening in the UK and beyond.

During the furore over whether or not we should be heading for a single European currency, I was paying a visit to the European Parliament to take part in a conference on the future of health services and the role of trades unions. During the journey I chanced across a copy of *Europa Times*. The banner headline? 'German poll shows only 23% in favour of European currency'. Suddenly I didn't feel so bad about being a Eurosceptic! Find out what other people think.

What magazines do you read?

Make sure you read (and write for), your 'trade' magazine. More important read magazines about things you don't understand! If you haven't caught on to the fact that computers and computing are going to change your life forever then this book has been a wasted journey. If you are not a computer type, you can be and must be. Try any of the computer magazines with the acronym 'PC' in its title.

What else? You will find amazing the number of businesses and industries that are struggling with the same problems you are. They may call them something different but the nub of the problem will be the same. The solutions may be different and with any luck, may just be innovative enough to give you a new slant on what you can do.

Hospitals are worrying about closures, mergers and down-sizing; highstreet retailers are worrying about big name shops moving out of town. Solutions are similar. One hospital chairman lived in an area where M&S had established an edge-of-town store. To save the high street and smaller shops, M&S were persuaded to establish a park and ride scheme to bus shoppers to and from the town centre, to and from the edge-of-town store. My chairman friend pinched the idea and established a hospital bus service to bring patients from outlying areas into the hospital and then to the town, to do their shopping. The buses are always packed.

What TV news programmes do you watch?

I watch them all! Including cable news network (CNN). The message is the same one I gave you in the newspaper section (page 141). Get an alternative, outside perspective. If it does nothing else it will remind you how good the BBC is!

When did you last learn something?

Go on a course, join a night school, holiday programme – sure if you want to, great idea. But how about learning something from someone you work with? The chances are you work in an invisible university and haven't realized it. Unipart has turned its business into a university. Its aim is to improve staff skills and make and sell things that are better because of it. Unipart is worth a visit – you might learn something!

Can you type?

Learn! Keyboards are here for a while yet.

My mother is 75 years old – please don't tell her I told you. For her last birthday we took her to France by Le Shuttle. Turn up, buy a ticket and put the car on a train. Thirty-five minutes later, we are in Calais and ready for lunch. That's the theory.

What really happens? Turn up, get the ticket – OK, so far. Try and board the train and you wait in an eighty-car queue, with engine running, cursing; whilst a French gendarme or border person, transcribes the names of the travellers from their passports into a computer. The trouble is – he can't type.

So, we all sit in our queue, whilst Monsieur Dactylo does a Woody Woodpecker impression on the keyboard of his computer, tapping one letter at a time. I have lost track of the amount of cash it took to dig the hole and run the rails. I think the company have to find about £10 million a day just to service their borrowings. They seem to have overlooked the fact that, Monsieur Woodpecker is stuffing the business down a quite different hole!

Never mind bar code technology, or swiping the passports through a reader. Never mind we are all in this tangle called the European Union and we are not supposed to need all this stuff any more. Just teach this man to type, or get a secretary, or some one who can. Right now, a computer means a keyboard – so type!

Do computers frighten you, or excite you?

No goose bumps – no future. Nothing else to say.

How many holidays do you take?

Take as many as you can. Holidays are a great way of staying in shape. Because...

What you do on holiday

...matters!

Take a break, get a tan, do all that stuff but take one day to learn something. In the NHS, whether you are going on holiday to Barbados, Benidorm or Bognor Regis; drop a note to your counterpart in the local hospital and pay a visit. Not only will you be welcomed, but you will see how other people do a job similar to yours. Work in a factory, laboratory, shop or whatever, drop a note, pay a visit. Holiday learning, makes friends, encourages exchange and increases understanding.

Futureproof yourself by becoming a resource centre. A library of knowledge, a flexible friend and an asset.

Soft in the middle?

Organizations that are **Futureproofed** have a rule. The rule is:

'if it don't add value, we ain't gonna do it'.

A product or service is not going to be enough. A service has got to have brains, too. Hospital managers don't realize out-patient clinics that are clean and friendly, efficient and run on time are not good enough. They are providing services without brains. A service with brains recognizes out-patients often include people who work, have kids, household responsibilities, or are elderly. Services that start at nine in the morning making mum drag two kids on to the bus in the middle of the rush hour, or force an elderly person to the end of a rush hour bus queue, are services without brains. Out-patient clinics held early in the afternoon or in the evening mean easier travel, less time taken off work and are smart — they have brains!

Washing machine repair companies that send out repair mechanics during the day, Monday to Friday only; overlook the huge percentage of women who work. (We would do well to remember; 36% of women between the ages of 16 and 59, work full time and have children. 29% work part-time. If that is not what's called having your hands full I don't know what is!) Good mechanics — lousy, brain-dead services.

Brain-dead services don't add value. Smart services have value +**Plus**.

Here is a value +**Plus** service. Do you have a car? Does it need servicing?

We will pick up your car at about 8.30pm, when you get home. We will then service it overnight, valet it and bring it back during the night to your home, pop the keys through the letter box and leave a copy of the *Wall Street Journal* (OK, OK, *The Telegraph* or the *Sun* or the *Guardian* or whatever), on the seat. Payment is by credit card over the 'phone.

The service is cheaper because the garage is using its fixed overhead 24hrs a day and faster because there is nothing on the roads at 3am.
Smart services have value *+Plus*. These services break down ordinary business processes. They break out of the boxes that businesses come in. Processes become continuums. Rover has broken up not just its business but all its suppliers too. It has 'smart services have value *+Plus*' and just-in-time delivery. I'm not talking conventional just-in-time. This is 'smart services have value *+Plus*' and just-in-the-nick-of-time delivery. It services its running line, (its production line), every fifteen minutes! Its production facility is designed around 'just-in-the-nick-of-time'.

The people

That's the services, the business, now what about the people? Let's talk about the film industry. Huge complex movies are made by people who are hired to do a job, do it and leave. The building industry is populated by an army of self-employed skills specialists who do their bit and go. These people add value to a movie or a building and are gone before they add costs. A complex network of people, picked for their skills and experience, is drawn together. The people are put to work and are gone when their work is done. People who may have never worked together before, work for each other as part of a team.

Futureproofing tells us skills are the passport to security and organizations will look very different in the future. People who take charge of their skills and development will **Futureproof** themselves and their fortunes. Work is set to look very different.

Sits-vac'

Knowledge-based workers

who add value

please apply here!

The invisible organization

Technology makes businesses shrink, it's as simple as that. Jobs done with fewer people, better. No armies of staff to house, feed and water and buildings get smaller. People who are 'out-there' doing the business and who don't need to 'come here', means 'here' becomes a different place.

Banks are learning. Customers don't find it funny to risk parking on a double yellow line, fight their way through the high street, queue up at the counter and beg to see the bank manager. Or, be assailed by a complete stranger, a third of their age, and be told that they 'are their personal banker'.

Banks are learning: picking up a 'phone, pressing a few numbers to deal with the every day business and having the manager come to see you, is a much better deal. The bank becomes invisible – popping up wherever it's needed. All companies are at the end of a 'phone, like the pizza delivery company.

Futureproofed businesses will be invisible and come to you when you call. Property is an asset the value of which can go down as well as up. Why take the risk? Turn the high street banks into burger bars whilst you still can. If you have to be in a property, rent it and walk away when it is too small, or too big or too anything that you don't want anymore.

Government should not own a single brick. Hospitals should be in rented offices, converted into hospitals for the duration. In the last ten years bed-stays have fallen from ten days to six and a half days. Technology will drive that figure further down. Why have the expense of capital costs hanging around the neck of the tax payer? This goes for any business. Shareholders are no different. If the shape of your business has changed over the last ten years, you can bet the changes will compound in the next five.

What can the government do for you?

You must know the joke? There are three lies in business. 'I will buy one from you tomorrow, the cheque is in the post and I am from the government and I want to help you.'

The joke is they do! Governments want to do popular things. I'm not talking politics, I'm talking government. Governments need to do popular things. The problem is there is not a lot left they can do that is popular. Cutting taxes means reducing services. Popular with the minority who are fit and wealthy. Unpopular with the majority who are not – and that is where the votes are. That is the crux of the problem.

Small grants to get businesses started encourage sloppy management and encourage demands for more help later. Greenhouse plants seldom do well in a frost.

Restrictive education systems modelled around a syllabus designed to meet a national objective may teach kids to appreciate poetry but may not be best suited to helping your son or daughter to learn to spell. Educational achievement is all about average passes. Averages can move down as well as up. If you have the chance, make sure your child is educated in more than one country. Think about an overseas university to follow a normal degree course.

Health services that argue with social services about what is social care and what is health care, may protect an income tax budget from a community tax budget, but do 'something-all' for granny – who just needs a bit of help.

The whole dreariness of it all drags on and on. How do we **Futureproof** ourselves?

Steer clear of government! Watch them like a hawk and make contact with your MP as often as you can! The only ways government can please are to cut taxes and spend more money – it can't be done.

Don't rely on currency to make a profit and always expect currency to move in the wrong direction. Insulate your export sales against the movement of currency and never, never, never ever take a chance on a currency. Freddy Laker would still be in business, carting holiday makers off to the sun, if he had watched out for that piece of advice. He borrowed money in dollars and paid it back in pounds. Great idea until the currency values shifted.

Don't expect government agencies to perform, they can't. They are strangled by a system that rewards safety and punishes risk taking. Politics is about safe decisions and getting re-elected.

As the Police Force (no damn it, I will have my way), service are swamped with more drugs-related crimes they will be forced to ignore all avoidable property crime. That is why a MINTEL report, as long ago as 1989 predicted security would be in the top three growth businesses of the decade. They are right. Private security firms will flourish.

The NHS is bound to collapse. Technology and expectations are driving it further and further along a journey from which there is no return. Both political parties want it to survive – it can't. Get healthy and stay that way!

Fears about the welfare and health of the growing elderly population are probably overstated. Alzheimer's disease and all of those wretched illnesses are a rich vein for pharmaceutical companies. Drugs to deal with dementia will be in place in the next five years. There is just too much money in it for the pharmaceutical boys not to be up to their armpits in secret development – right now!

Don't expect private medicine to come to the rescue. Private medical insurance is a risk. The firms that offer the services are as beset with problems as their nationalized counterparts. Problems such as higher expectations, greater costs forced by technological advances and fewer people in the sort of employment well enough off, to be able to pay the premiums. Many will be driven out of business.

Private medicine is a mug's game. Most premium payers are economically active upper middle class, white collar working men and women between 25 and 55 years old. It is at this time of their lives that people need health care the least. Average, full-cover premiums are running at about £900 per year. Total payments over thirty years £27 000 – nice business. A bookmaker would turn green.

The future is in the privatization of the NHS. A political time bomb and poll tax in bandages. The service could remain free at the point of delivery, funded by tax pounds, it will just be run by people who know what they are doing without the costs of government on their backs.

Futureproofing is insulation. Welfare is wealth.

Final word

The final word is Rupert Murdock's, not mine. Whilst writing this book I watched a TV programme about him. A smarty-type interviewer was hectoring him about the size of his empire, his dominance of the media and the size of his market share (he says 10.8% of UK media).

Murdock looked irritated, he'd had enough of this.

> 'Look', he said, 'Anyone could have started Sky television. Anyone could have revolutionized the UK newspaper industry. You lot sat on your backsides and I did it'.

That's ***Futureproofing***!

Things to stay awake and worry about

> No one ever became a success by losing sleep and worrying about things – the way to be a success is to get someone else to lay awake and worry.
> *I can't remember where I pinched this from, but I just love it – wicked isn't it!*

- Write down five ways to sustain competitive advantage.

- How do you know you're any good? Name three organizations you could 'benchmark' with.

- Now name two, outside your industry, that you could benchmark with.

- Set a date by which time you will have it set up.

- What percentage of your turnover do you commit to training?

- What is your industry norm? Double it in your next budget.

- What percentage of your turnover do you commit to information technology?

- What is your industry norm? Double it in your next budget.

- How do you influence culture in your organization?

- How many of your staff do you know by name?

- What percentage of your time do you spend walking about in the organization? Double it!

- Do you usually:
  - memo people?
  - phone them and tell them what you want?
  - go and see them?

- Have you identified your successor?

- Who is it?

- Can you do more with:
  - fewer people?
  - a smaller budget?
  - in a shorter time cycle?

No? Think again, you're going to have to, your competitors will.

Organizing propositions

Do you think the following statements are true? Use them as discussion points with colleagues and staff.

- Public services will be 'enabled', that is not carried out by the organizations themselves, but carried out under contract.

- Business processes will give way to 'horizontal continuums'.

- Better work is done in teams.

- Individual contributions in teams will become more important and not be dependent on seniority or status.

- Staff will invest in their own skills.

- The customer will be the boss.

- There will be constant reorganization around the customer's vision.

- Information technology will be everything.
- There will be no 'new address'.
- Organizations are only concepts.

Epilogue

In the end, there is just a new beginning

When we've finished frightening ourselves to death with the spectre of what's to come – there is still tomorrow. We know governments have an appetite for our money and for lying to us about what they do with it. We know our state-run services are trapped in administrative slums and grinding to a halt. We know we are not educating our kids enough (let alone the adults). We know we pay people not to work. We know we are at the beginning of a technological revolution that will eclipse everything we've so far seen.

Well, at least we know. We can't say no one told us, we couldn't have known, there was no way we could have found out. The facts are like a big red bus careering driverless down the high street – a disaster waiting to happen.

But we still have to survive. We will do it by running our organizations in new ways, creating stability from change. Creating work and wealth by competing and being better at what we do than our neighbours. By understanding what the 14 year olds are learning for their GCSEs by 'developing a knowledge and understanding of the environment within which business activity takes place and the way in which changes in that environment influence business behaviour'.

The opening paragraph of Will Hutton's *The State We Are In* (Random House, 1995) is too tempting not to repeat here.

The British are accustomed to success. This is the world's oldest democracy.

> Britain built an Empire, launched the Industrial Revolution and was on the winning side in the twentieth century's two world wars. The British believe their civilisation is admired all over the world. A Briton does not boast openly, but is possessed of an inner faith that he or she is special. To be born in these islands is still seen as a privilege.

He doesn't think we can live up to these ideals. I do, if we **Futureproof**.

You must read

Hutton, W (1995) *The State We Are In*, Random House.

Kennedy, P (1993) *Preparing for the Twenty First Century*, HarperCollins.

Hamel, G and Prahalad, CK (1994) *Competing for the Future*, Harvard Business School Press.

Kissinger, H (1994) *Diplomacy*, Simon & Schuster.

The Report of the Commission for Social Justice (1994) Vintage.

The *Harvard Business Review*.

The *European* newspaper.

The *Wall Street Journal*.

Any (or all) of the PC magazines.

Business and Technology magazine.

Computer Weekly.

Anything by Tom Peters.

Everything by Edward de Bono.

Stop press

Who's who?

Do you know who you are? Or, should I say what you are? Because no one else does! Who you are and what you do is important. It is important to you and yours. It is also important to lots of other people. Who you are and what you do places you somewhere in the Government's Social Class Classifications.

The classifications were first devised in 1911, to explain variations in death rates. By 1921 the breakdowns had been refined to their present form and were based on an estimate of the skill that was required to do a particular job.

The social class breakdown was devised in the days when families consisted of a mum and a dad, under one roof, with dad the breadwinner and mum a housewife. How things have changed. The problem is the Social Class Register hasn't.

The current definitions are 70 years old and the definitions of occupations exclude 40% of the population. Yes, 40%. Those not on the list include housewives, the long-term sick and the growing numbers not in employment. Note, not 'unemployed' but, 'not in employment' and we know there is a world of difference. Within these groups are some of society's most disadvantaged groups.

The explosion of women's employment, contract working, self-employment and part-time working has become impossible to classify under the old system. The definitions are riddled with anomalies. For example the high-powered secretary to the boss of an international conglomerate, a public company is in the same social class as a petrol pump attendant or the junior in the typing pool.

Does it matter? Yes, it sure does! Not just to the manufacturers of products who want to target their resources and develop the products that we want. Important though that is, it is not the main point. The crucial point is the definitions are also used for scientific and medical research and the allocation of government money. Given the pressures that we know exist on health, welfare and social services – how much money and resource have gone in the wrong direction because the decisions are based on incorrect data?

All this came to light days before this book **Futureproofing** was to be printed. Thanks to modern technology, last minute additions to a book are less of a headache than they used to be. Nevertheless it was a close-run thing. I thought it was important to add this news to the book, because, at least, now we know and thank goodness it is to change – but not for a while.

The Office of Population Censuses and Surveys has commissioned work to look into the mess. The Economic and Social Research Council will be producing more robust definitions and as a result we should get better policies and more accurate market research. The bad news is, the work is to be completed in time for the 2001 census – years away.

The new definitions will have to be 'backward looking' insofar as they need to reflect the way in which data have been captured in the past, otherwise there will be no way of detecting long-term trends. This is vital for epidemiologists, for example.

However a system that has three classifications for farm workers, who are now only 2% of the population and just one for junior, non-manual workers who are 20%, needs a good sort out.

Futureproofing is tricky enough, without having to make do with clapped-out data. Remember, there are lies, damned lies and some 50 year old definitions. You have been warned!

APPENDIX: **Give us this day our daily bread**

The chart on the following page follows the development of one of the greatest companies of the post-war world – from a garage to the space age in about 7500 days. The development of Microsoft and their products, taken as a case study of corporate development is impressive enough. More important, perhaps sinister, is the influence the Company's products has over our daily lives.

The development of the Microsoft DOS platform is the foundation of most of the computer systems we use today. The Windows operating system is now an industry standard. There are few products and services that we use and enjoy that do not, in some way, reach us, care of a computer and a Microsoft product.

The size of the market share, the influence of the product and the power Microsoft has over our daily lives are awesome, overwhelming, monumental, and terrifying. And, they've made a pile of bread for themselves and their shareholders!

I visited a factory that makes bread. I met a man who introduced me to the mixer of the ingredients, the controller of the portions, the supervisor of the baking time and the energy conservation, the re-orderer of ingredients, the invoicer of the customers, the superintendent of the delivery schedules and the authorizer of the wages. It was a computer.

What have you been doing in the last 20 years?

January 1975	*Inspired by an article in Popular Electronics about the MITS Altaria 8800 minicomputer, Paul Allen and Bill Gates formed Microsoft and developed a version of BASIC, a computer language, for the machine. They wrote it and sold it to MITS in one month*
July 1977	*Microsoft develops a second computer language product FORTRAN*
December 1979	*By the end of the year Microsoft sales exceed US$1 million*
June 1981	*Microsoft reorganize themselves into a privately held corporation, with Bill Gates as the Chairman of the Board and President and Paul Allen as executive vice president*
August 1981	*IBM introduces a personal computer with Microsoft's MS-DOS software as its basis*
March 1982	*The first UK subsidiary of Microsoft is established*
April 1983	*Microsoft develop the 'mouse'*
September 1983	*'Word', Microsoft's word processing package is launched*
November 1983	*'Windows' is launched*
May 1984	*Microsoft launch a software developer's tool-kit to make writing programmes for Windows easier for independent developers*
August 1985	*Sales top US$140 million*
March 1986	*Microsoft go public and a US$1 share becomes worth US$28 in one day*
April 1987	*Microsoft and IBM operate a joint operating system called OS/2*
January 1988	*Based on sales, Microsoft becomes the world leading software company*
June 1989	*Microsoft launches its 'multi-media' division*
May 1990	*Microsoft sales top US$1.2 billion*
April 1992	*Windows version 3.1 is launched with advanced orders of over one million copies*
October 1992	*Windows for Workgroups is launched*
January 1993	*Based on stock value, Microsoft becomes the largest company in the computer industry*
March 1993	*MS-DOS version six is on sale*
May 1993	*Windows upgrade NT is launched*
June 1994	*New version Windows '95 on test*

Continued

October 1994	*Microsoft and computer company Intuit announce their intention to merge*
May 1995	*Microsoft pulls out of Intuit deal, fearing anti-competition intervention by the US Justice Department*

(Source: Computing Weekly, *June 29, 1995.)*

Index

Figures and Tables are indicated by *italic page numbers*